Hello Beautiful
All-Natural Face and Skin Care

200+ Step-by-Step Photos In This Skin Care Book

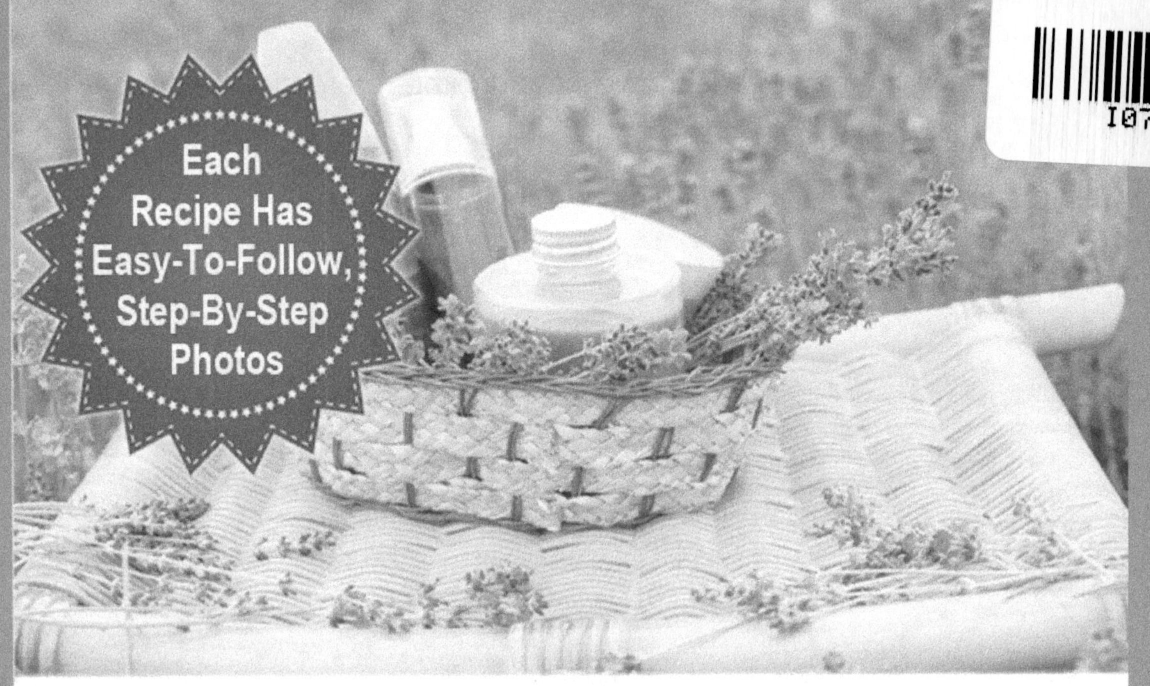

Learn How To Make Easy Lotions, Scrubs, Sunscreen, Moisturizers and More...

2nd Edition
Melinda Niles

Disclaimer

The author disclaims any personal liability, for loss or risk incurred as a result of any information or advice contained herein, either directly or indirectly.

All links are for informational purposes only and are not warranted for content, accuracy, or other implied or explicit purposes. All links were working at the time of this eBook's release but may now have expired.

The author does not intend to render health, wellness or other professional advice in the documents contained herein. The reader is encouraged to seek competent health and wellness advice before engaging in any activity in this book.

Contents

Introduction

Face care is one of the most important aspects of any beauty routine. However, most people make the mistake of using over the counter products to cleanse, tone and scrub their face. These products are loaded with harmful chemicals, can lead to many unwanted side effects and can even damage the skin.

Fortunately, there is a solution that allows you to beautify and nourish your face without exposing it to any of the dangerous chemicals in conventional beauty products. In addition, to natural face care, I've included tutorials for:

- Natural sunscreen – Reducing sun damage keeps your skin looking young
- Natural insect repellent – Keeping insects away keeps your skin healthy
- Air cleansing plants – Keeping your air clean keeps your face and skin healthy
- And more ways to keep your skin and face radiant

For each natural tutorial, you get:
- A list of the required ingredients
- Step by step text instructions that explain how to prepare the face cleansers, mask or scrub
- Supporting photographs that show the preparation steps

So, let's get started with these natural face care solutions!

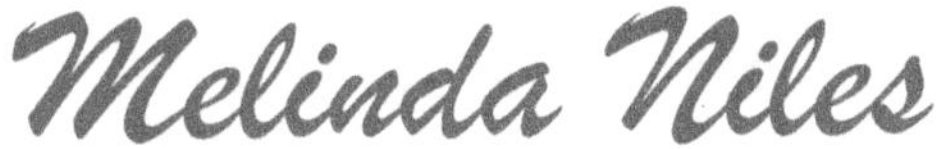

Cleansing Lotion for Sensitive Skin

Are you tired of trying all the cleansing lotions on Earth and not being satisfied by any of them? Are you very busy and you don't have the time to go to the store to buy some cleansing milk? Do you want to use only natural ingredients for your skin?

Then, it is time to start preparing your own cosmetic products. They are a lot cheaper, a lot healthier and you can use a lot of ingredients from your own kitchen.

What You'll Need:

- ✓ 1/2 cup oat flakes
- ✓ 1/2 cup filtered water
- ✓ 1 tsp sweet almond oil
- ✓ 1/2 tbsp sour cream

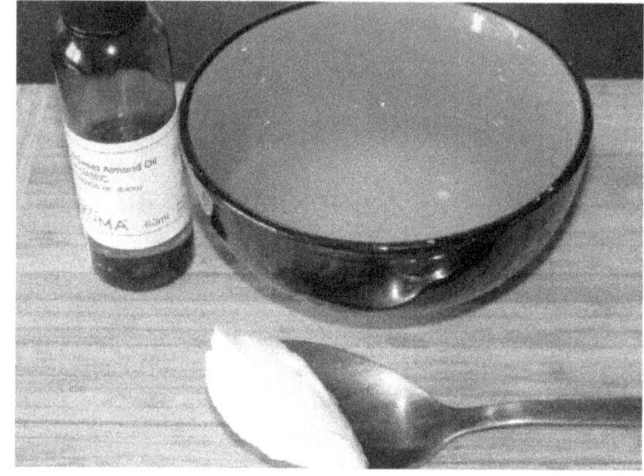

Directions:

1. Pour the water into a pan and bring it to a boil. When the water starts to boil, decrease the heat to low.

2. Add the oat flakes and let them boil for 10 minutes. If the mixture is too thick, pour one or two tablespoons of filtered water.

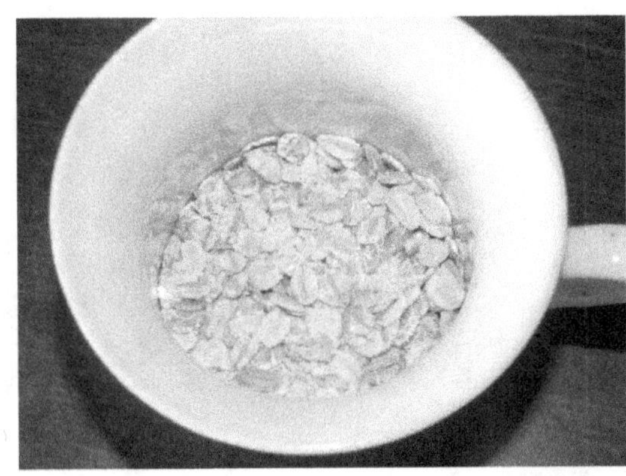
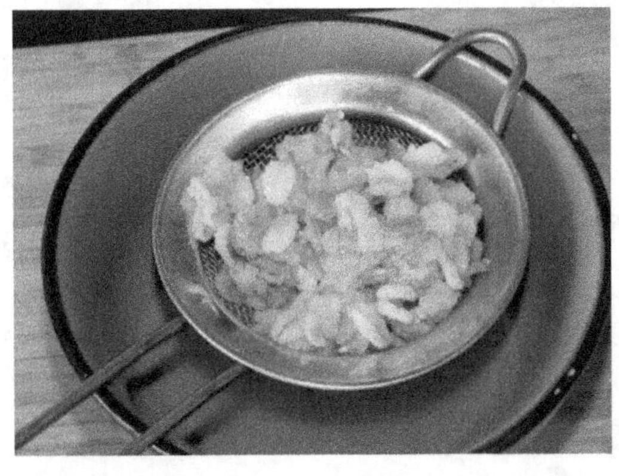
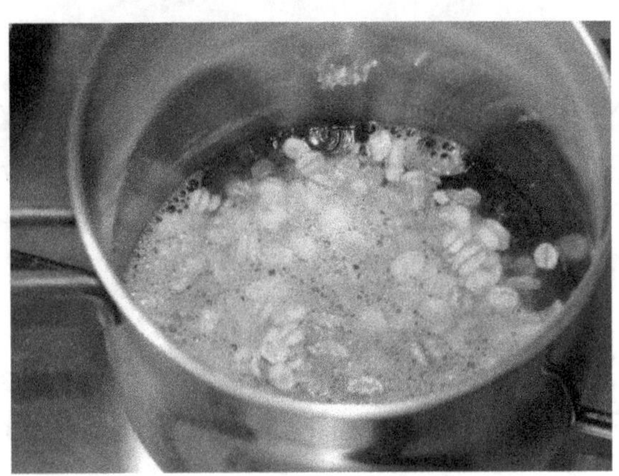

3. Remove from heat and let it cool, then drain the liquid.

4. Add the sour cream and oil and mix well.

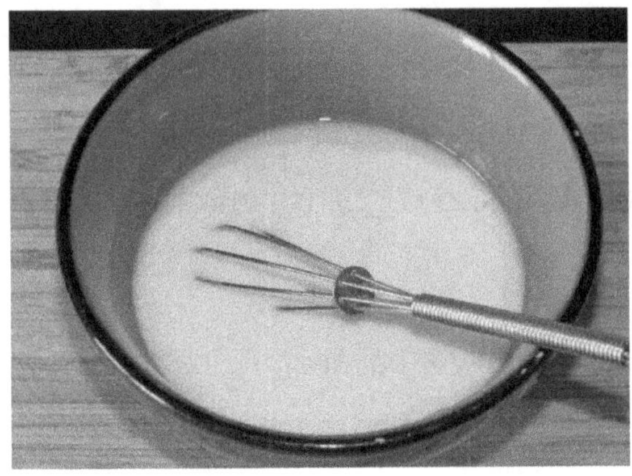

5. Use a container with a lid for storage.

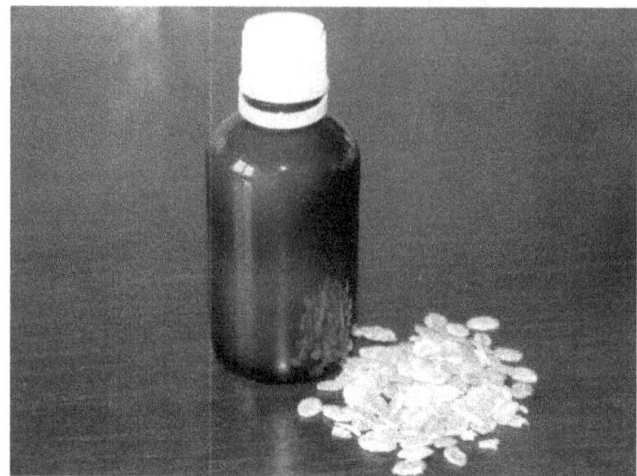

6. Keep the lotion in the fridge for 3-4 days.
7. Shake well before each use and apply with a cotton pad.

Cocoa and Coffee Facial Mask

I just love the smell of fresh ground coffee and the taste of chocolate. Well, who doesn't? I read somewhere that chocolate comes from cocoa, which is a tree, that makes it a plant. Therefore, chocolate counts as salad. I rest my case :)

Besides the great, unique taste, cocoa has a lot of benefits for internal and skin health. It contains many antioxidants that fight free radicals and has rejuvenation and anti-aging properties.

In its raw state, cocoa has more compounds that lead to the wellbeing of the body: arginine is a natural aphrodisiac, anandamide is a substance that causes a state of euphoria, tryptophan serves as an antidepressant. It also contains neurotransmitters that stimulate and balance the brain activity.

Epicatecina-galato, a compound found in cocoa, actually a flavanol, helps to increase the relaxation capacity of the blood vessels. It is also found in red wine, green tea and grapefruit juice, all of them recommended for preventing heart disease and keeping cholesterol under control. Also, cocoa is rich in magnesium, which helps the heart to pump blood more efficiently, strengthens bones and lowers blood pressure. Maybe because of magnesium, a mineral with calming properties, craving for chocolate is so common among women on their period.

Coffee is also good for your skin: it is a source of antioxidants as well; soothes the skin and brings back its glance; protects against sun rays; increases blood circulation.

What You'll Need:

- ✓ 4 tablespoons ground coffee
- ✓ 4 tablespoons raw cocoa powder
- ✓ 2 tablespoons honey
- ✓ 8 tablespoons whole milk

Directions:

1. Use a bowl to combine the cocoa powder and coffee.

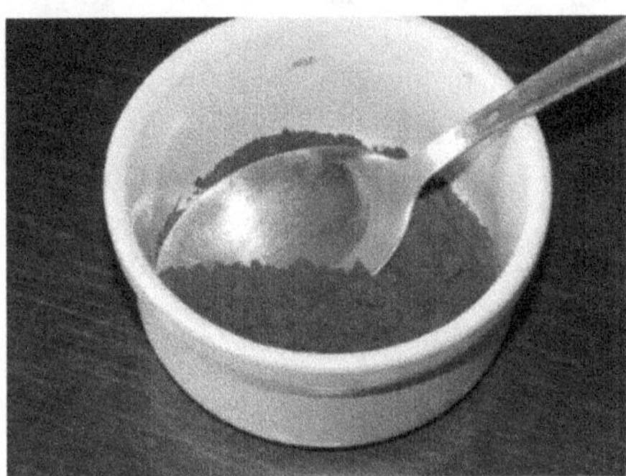

2. Pour the milk and mix well, then add the honey and mix again until well combined.

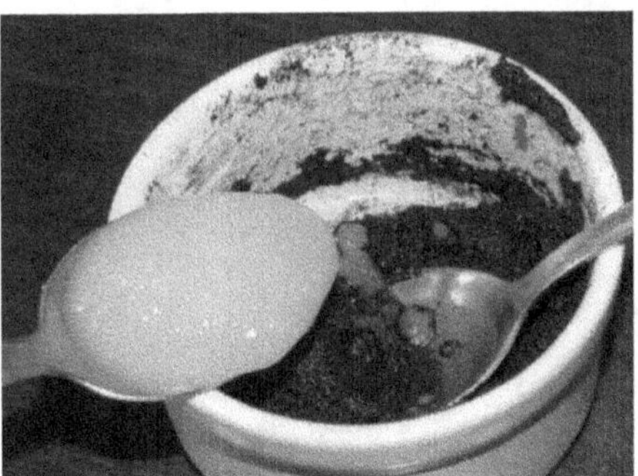

3. Apply the mixture to your skin and neck.

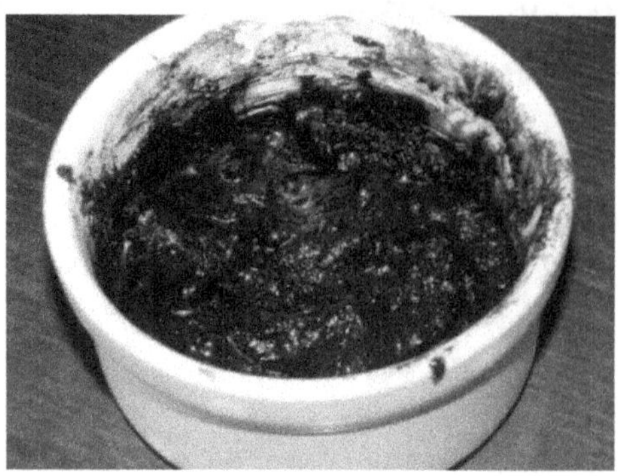

4. Leave it to dry.
5. Press a hot towel on to your face so the steam will soften the mask and it will be easier to remove.
6. Rinse well with warm water.
7. Apply a facial moisturizer.

Enjoy your soft and shiny skin!

If you want to start preparing homemade cosmetic products, you should know that some of them (especially the ones made from fruits and vegetables) have a short shelf life. For example, a facial cleansing lotion made with sour cream or buttermilk will last for no more than one week if you keep it in the fridge. This is due to the fact that it contains only natural ingredients and have no preservatives added.

This is a good thing because you know that no chemical or other synthetic substance will touch your face. However, sometimes you may like to have a facial cleanser that you can keep in your bathroom so you can use it anytime without having to go to the fridge to get it.

The below recipe contains natural ingredients and, in addition Vitamin E oil which is a natural preservative increases the shelf life of any cosmetic product.

What You'll Need:

- ✓ ¼ cup liquid baby soap/shampoo
- ✓ ¾ tsp avocado oil (or grape seed, sweet almond or even olive oil)
- ✓ ¼ cup boiling water
- ✓ 1 tbsp dried calendula flowers
- ✓ 8 drops essential oil (you will see below what kind of essential oil to use for your skin type)
- ✓ 6 drops (2 capsules) Vitamin E oil

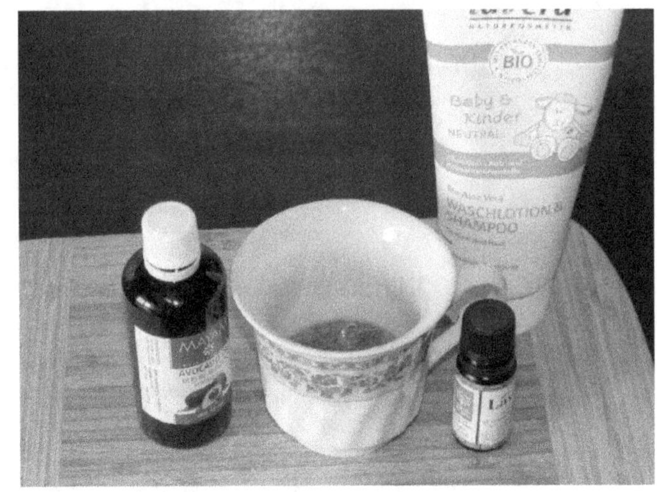

Directions:

1. Prepare an infusion by pouring the hot water over the calendula flowers.

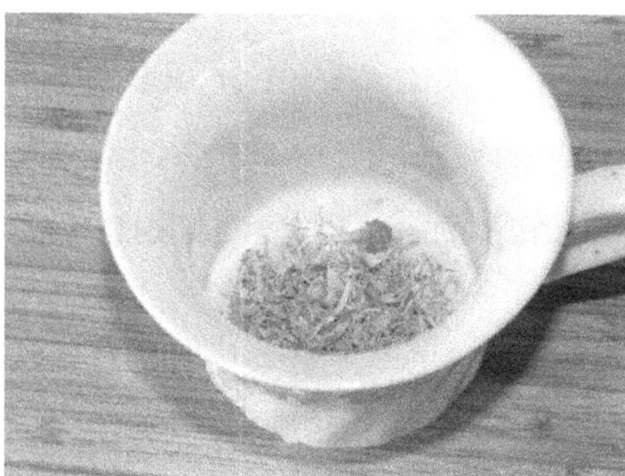 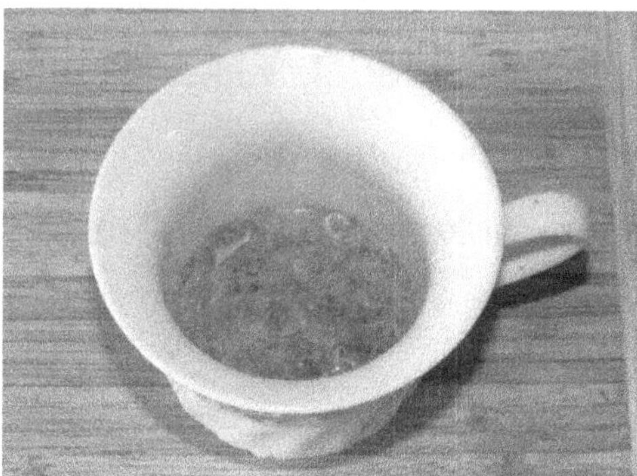

2. Let it cool.

3. Strain the liquid and set aside.

4. Combine the rest of the ingredients and mix them well.

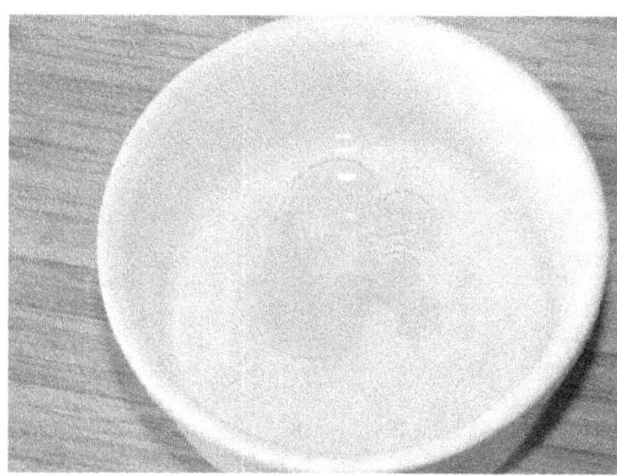 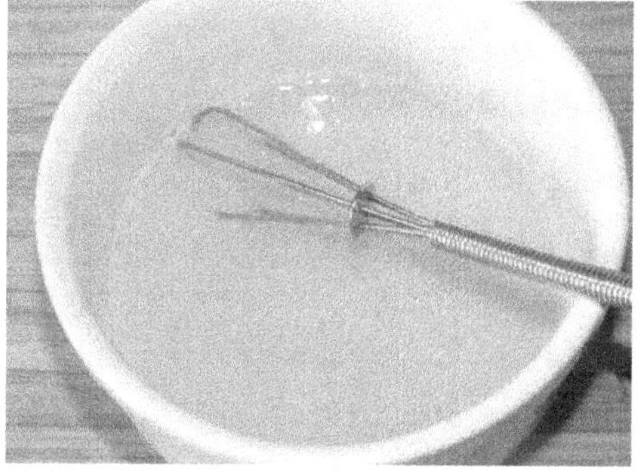

5. Add the calendula infusion and shake the container.

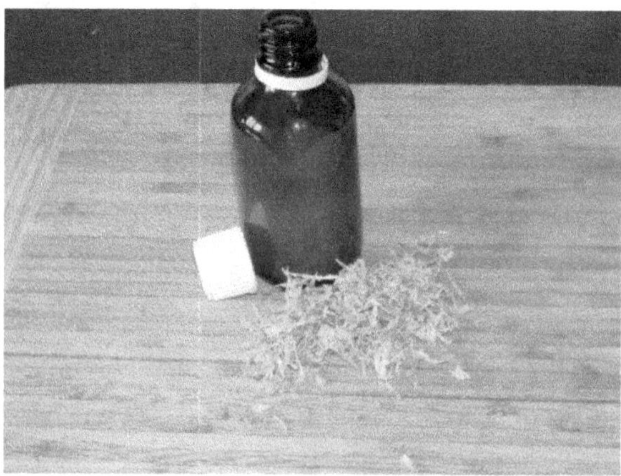

6. You may massage the cleanser with gentle moves on your face and neck or you can apply it by using a cotton pad.

7. Make sure you wash your face after using the cleanser, apply a toner and a moisturizer.

Which Essential Oil To Use?

- **For oily skin –** lemongrass, tea tree or geranium (they have an astringent effect).
- **For dry skin –** lavender, chamomile, rose or sandalwood.
- **For mature skin –** neroli, jasmine, lavender.
-

You can store this facial cleanser for a few weeks.

I really love simple recipes for homemade cosmetics that you can prepare yourself. Especially the ones with ingredients from my kitchen that don't make me run to the store to buy something so that I can get a specific lotion.

The below recipe enters this category and it is also very easy to make. You don't need fancy ingredients or some expensive equipment. Generally speaking, homemade cosmetics don't require exquisite stuff to get them done. Only a few natural ingredients, patience and the will to prepare them. And to use them, of course.

What You'll Need:

- ✓ ¼ cup dried elder flowers
- ✓ ½ cup boiling water
- ✓ ¼ cup buttermilk
- ✓ 1 tbsp honey

Directions:

1. Pour the hot water over the elder flowers and let steep until the mixture gets cool.

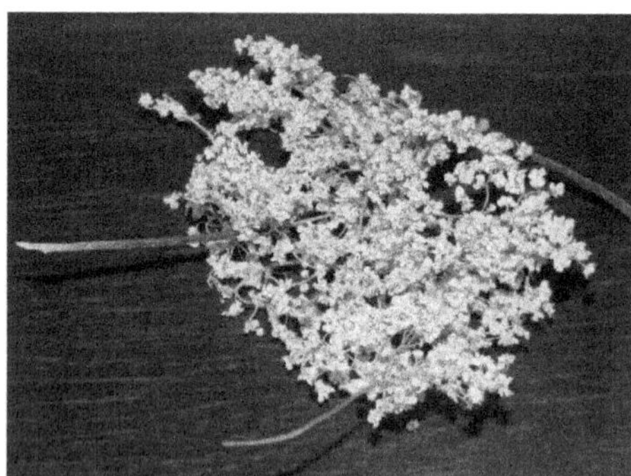 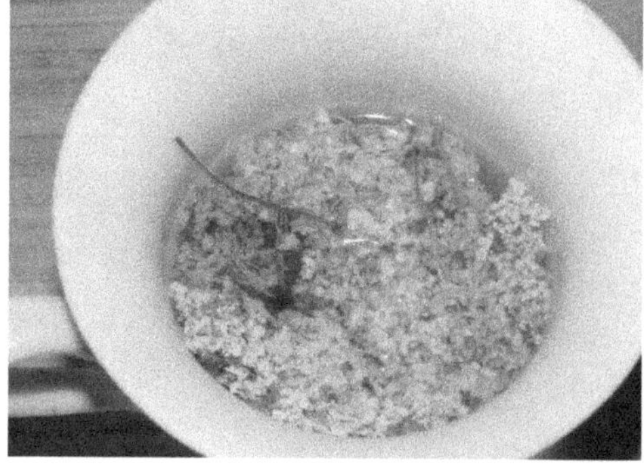

2. Strain the liquid through a cheesecloth.
3. Add the buttermilk and the honey and mix well.

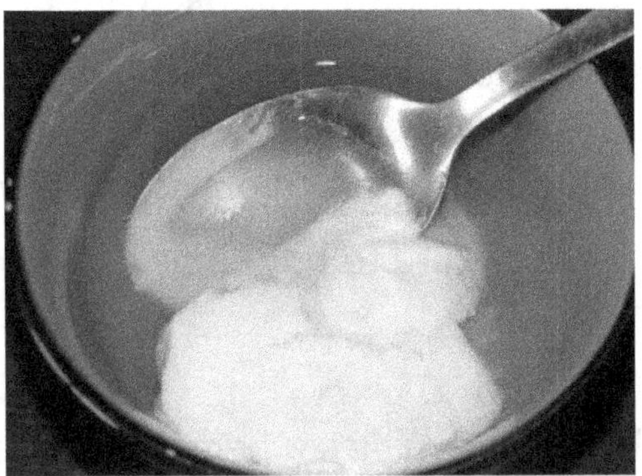 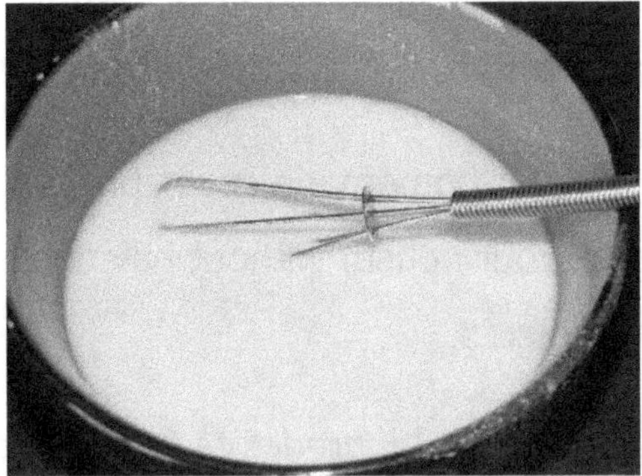

4. You can slightly massage your face and neck with the cleanser or you can use it on a cotton pad.
5. Rinse everything with warm water.
6. Store in the refrigerator for no more than 10 days.

My advice is to prepare smaller quantities so that the facial cleanser doesn't alter. The buttermilk is quite perishable and you should check the expiration date before you make the cleansing lotion.

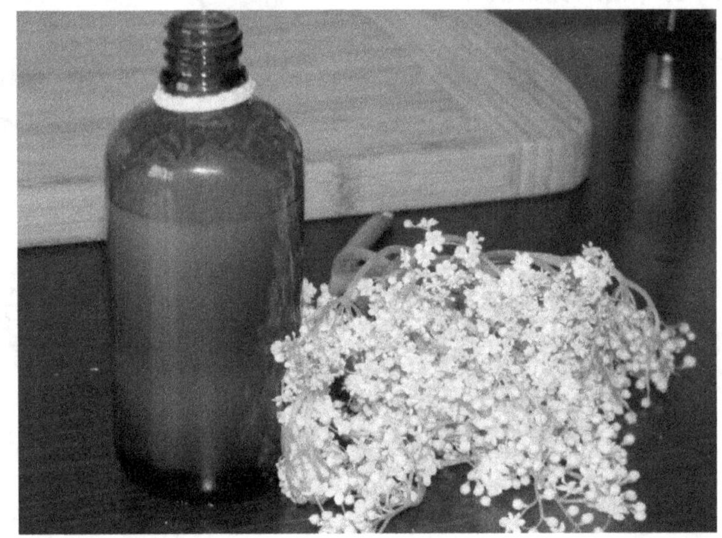

The mixture will leave your face clean and smooth.

You should use this cleanser twice a day on your beauty care routine. Follow it by applying a toner and your favorite homemade moisturizer.

The cleansing step should be present in our rituals everyday as there are a lot of impurities that remain stuck on our face and clog our pores. This may be one of the causes for premature aging of the skin.

As you know, your eyes and lips need cleansing too. It is important to take care of them and to use the same cleansing ritual that we have for the face.

The best part about homemade cosmetics is that you can use and combine anything you have inside your house, without having to run to the store to buy some expensive ingredients.

The recipe below uses 3 ingredients from my cupboard and makes a perfect cleanser for sensitive skin.

What You'll Need:

- ✓ 1 tablespoon calendula dried flowers
- ✓ ½ cup hot water
- ✓ 1 part oil (combination of sweet almond oil and Rosa Mosqueta oil)

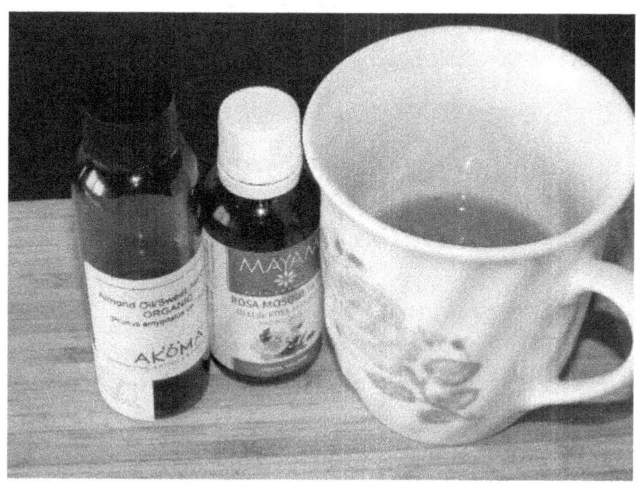

Directions:

1. Pour the hot water over the dried flowers and let steep for 10 minutes.

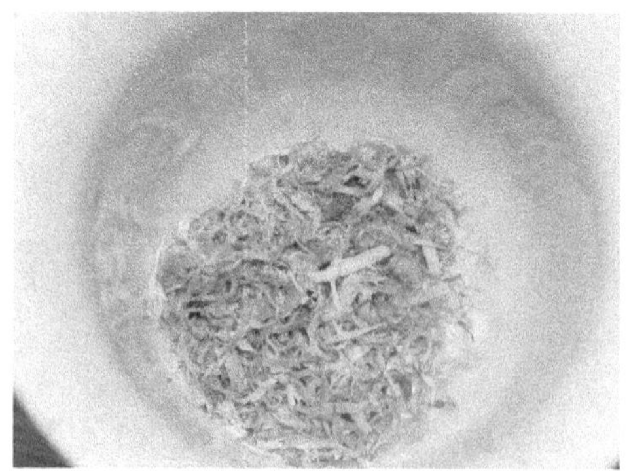
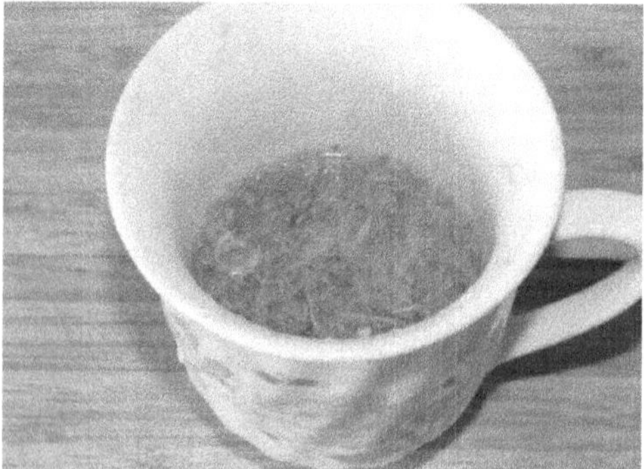

2. Drain the liquid and let it cool.

3. Use 1 part Infusion and 1 part oil combination.

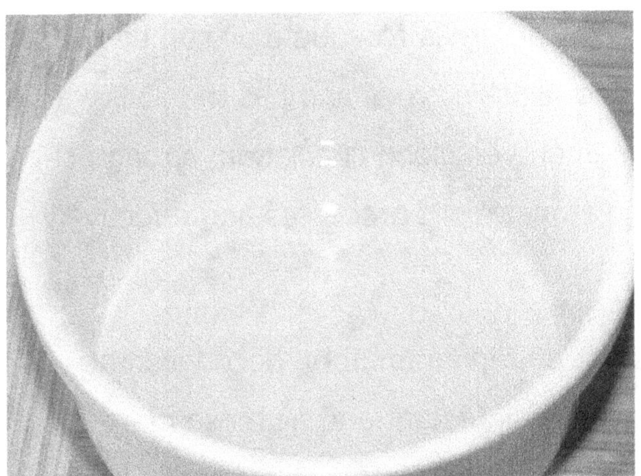

4. Place them in a dry container and shake well to mix.

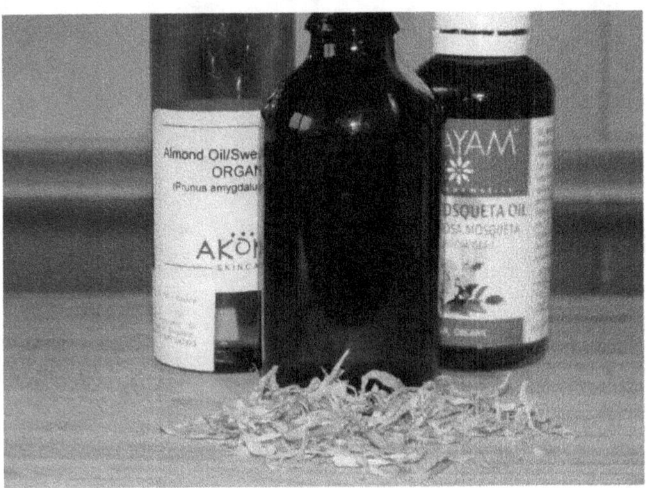

5. Use a cotton pad to remove the make-up and impurities from the eyes and lips.
6. You may also use this cleanser for your face and neck.
7. Store in the fridge for two weeks.
8. You may add 5-8 drops Vitamin E oil which is a natural preservative and will increase the cleanser's shelf life.

Calendula flowers contain colloidal silver which is a very effective antiseptic. In addition, they have a calming effect.

Almond oil is often used for cleansing even alone. Rosa Mosqueta oil can be used as a cleanser, but also for eyes. It is suitable for all skin types and has the ability to balance pH and vital functions of the skin, improves blood circulation, strong action of moisturizing the tissues, activating cellular metabolic processes and effectively combating free radicals.

It also presents the following characteristics: anti-inflammatory, decongestant, healing, antibacterial, antiviral, antiseptic and disinfectant and all those make it extremely useful for the various types of rashes, fungal infections, burns, scrapes or injuries. Its action is smooth and delicate and may be used even on the most sensitive skin like children's and infants'. Excellent results are obtained in the case of sensitive, dry, aging skin or cracked veins.

Honey Baking Soda Facial Scrub

I find the activity of preparing my own lotions and skin care products very pleasant and relaxing. It is so nice to combine all those natural ingredients in a way that will result in the best end product for my skin.

This happens because, throughout the years, I have discovered what is best for my skin. Beside the natural oils and butters, I use many herbs and also food ingredients from my kitchen.

This recipe has two such foods: baking soda and raw honey.

One of the ingredients always present in the kitchen, baking soda, invaded the cosmetic field. Its role in cosmetic treatments was first noticed by the Egyptians. Baking soda is a good facial scrub. It reduces redness and prevents the risk of pimples occurrence.

Raw honey has tremendous benefits for your skin health as well.

- It is suitable for all skin types, including sensitive skin.
- It acts as an antibacterial and anti-fungal agent, disinfecting the skin and fastens acne healing.
- Honey absorbs impurities and helps detoxify the skin.
- Is an excellent natural remedy for skin cleansing and toning.
- Softens and nourishes the skin, thanks to its emollient compounds.
- Is rich in antioxidants, which is why it restores the sun damaged skin and diminishes the fine lines.

That being said, I am confident that you will give this scrub a try.

What You'll Need:

- ✓ ½ tablespoon raw honey
- ✓ 1 tablespoon baking soda
- ✓ 1 drop frankincense essential oil
- ✓ 1 drop lavender essential oil
- ✓ 1 drop geranium essential oil

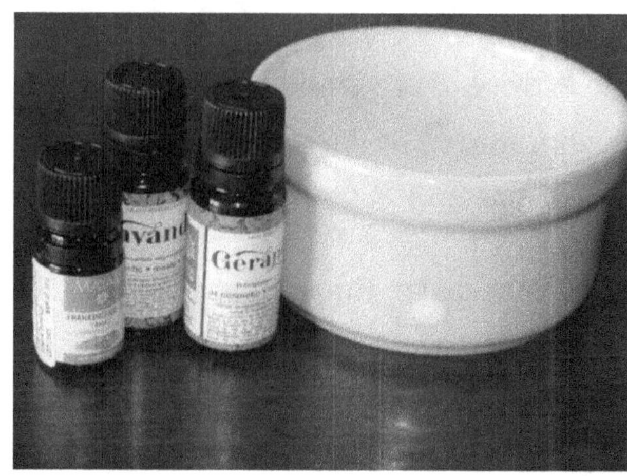

Directions:

1. Mix together the honey and the baking soda.

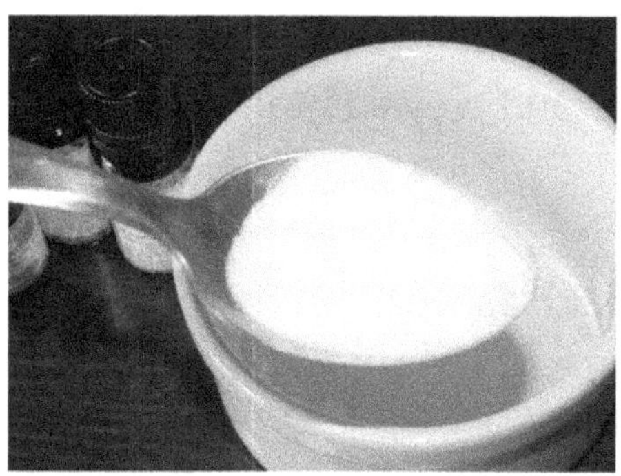
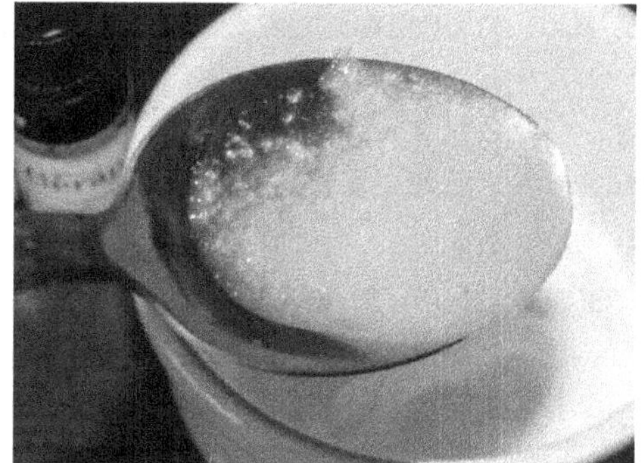

2. Add the essential oils.

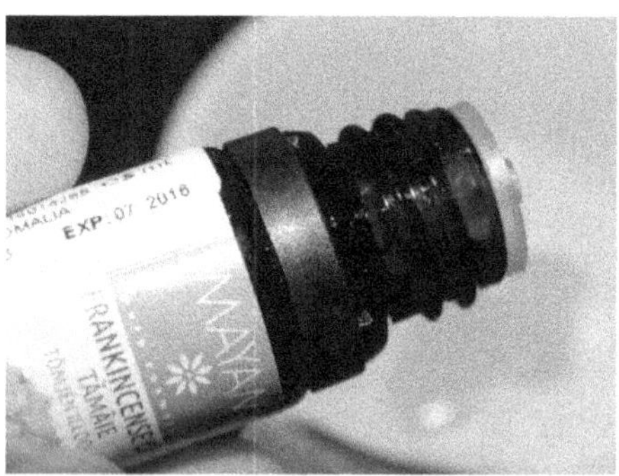
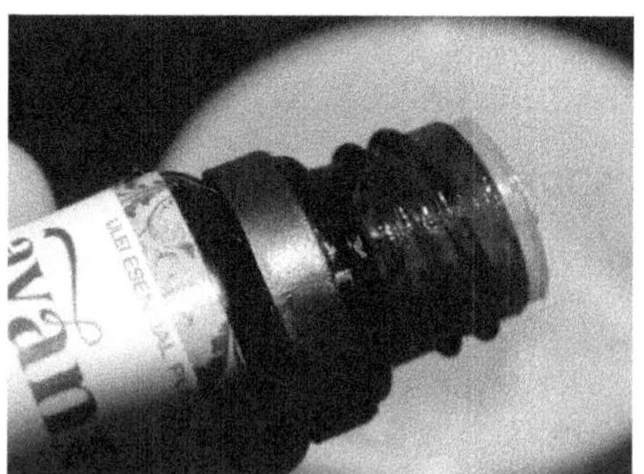

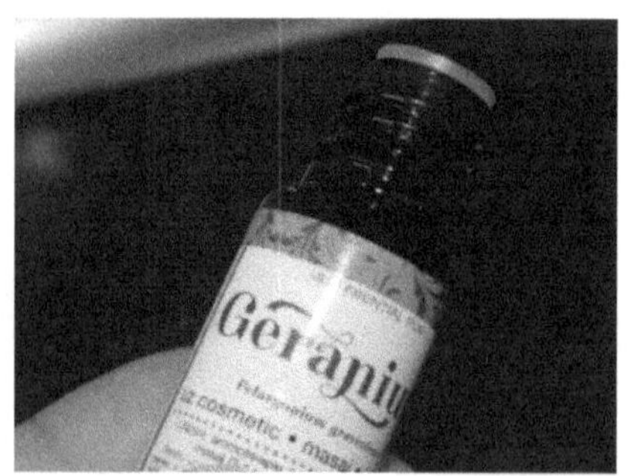

3. Take a warm towel and place it on your face. This will help open the pores.
4. Apply the scrub with gentle, circular moves. Massage the face for several minutes so that you remove all the impurities.
5. Wash the scrub with warm water.
6. Use it once/twice per week.

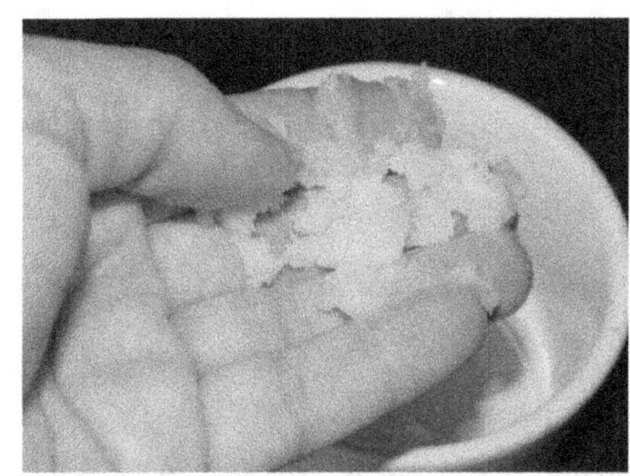

The pH of this scrub is alkaline, so if you want to balance it, sprinkle rose water on your face after you remove it.

Amongst the tropical fruits, kiwi can help you keep your skin young and healthy. You may do this either by eating it or by putting it on your face. How nice is that? I really like eating kiwi. And I don't seem to decide if I can spare a piece to create a face mask :)

If you usually don't have kiwi in your kitchen, here are the reasons to try it:

- **Rejuvenates skin -** it is a fruit that contains vitamins A, C and E. These vitamins are part of the antioxidants that are used in most cosmetic products. Vitamins A, C and E fight free radicals and maintain the beauty and elasticity of the skin. In addition, they help regenerate the collagen and maintain a firm foundation.
- **Reduces signs of aging -** regular consumption of kiwi can delay the signs of aging skin, wrinkles. It also successfully contributes to removing stains caused by the sun.
- **Helps detoxify the body -** in addition to the antioxidants, kiwi fruit is a rich source of dietary fiber, which helps eliminate toxins from the colon and thus detoxify the body. Your skin will look visibly healthier.
- **Helps healing -** being a fruit that is rich in vitamin C, regular consumption of kiwi fights inflammation and promotes collagen production. This way, cuts or other wounds will heal much faster. Furthermore, kiwi contains omega-3 fatty acids, compounds which prevent the development of skin diseases.
- **Fights against acne -** kiwi fruit pulp contains acids with anti-inflammatory properties that fight bacteria.
- **Other health effects -** regular consumption of kiwi fruit lowers the risk of respiratory disease, heart disease, colon cancer; lowers cholesterol levels.

Did I make my point? Are you willing to give it a try?

What You'll Need:

- ✓ 1 tablespoon sweet almond oil
- ✓ 2 tablespoons cane sugar
- ✓ ½ kiwi

Directions:

1. Mix together the oil and cane sugar.

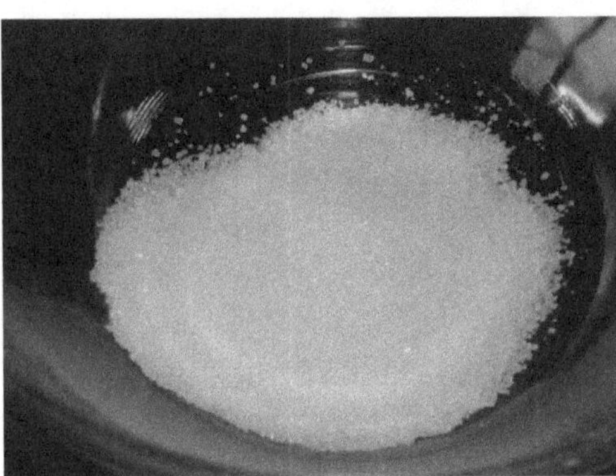 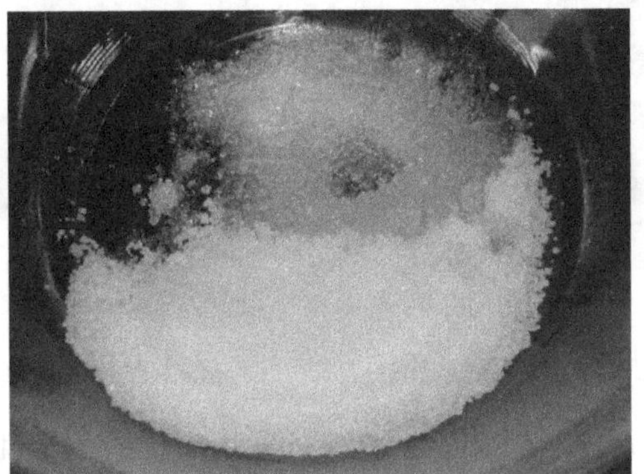

2. Chop the kiwi in very small pieces (avoid the core) and add it to the oil/sugar mixture.

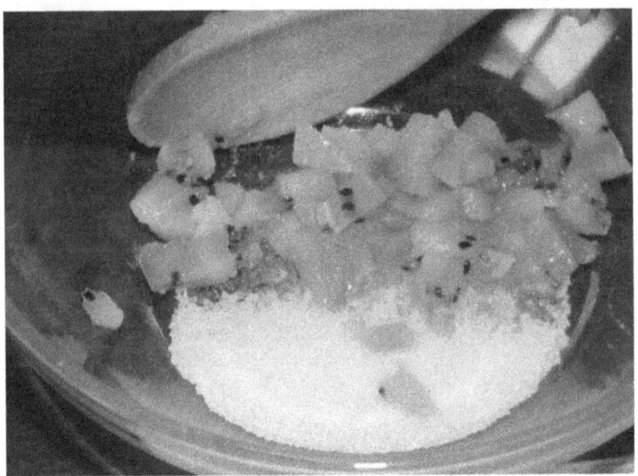

3. Mix well until you smash the fruit.

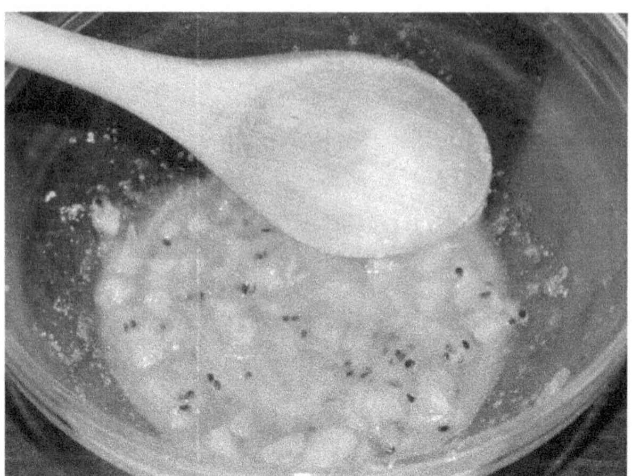

4. Apply with circular moves and massage the face and neck for at least 3 minutes. Allow the kiwi fruit to take action.
5. After that, rinse well with warm water and apply a face moisturizer.

You may keep the scrub in the fridge for two weeks.

Oatmeal Scrub for All Skin Types

I must confess that I love using face masks and scrubs. Although I usually don't have time to use them, I try to do my best. And when I get a spare moment, I pamper myself with face masks, body scrubs, homemade lotions so that it will be enough for the next month or so. Obviously it is not enough but, as I said, I do my best.

The recipe below uses some common, non-expensive ingredients which are great for the health of your skin. It is suitable for all skin types.

- **Oatmeal –** the flakes reduce skin irritation and inflammation. Also, oatmeal contains saponins, which are responsible for deeply cleaning the skin. It is very helpful in treating acne.
- **Brown sugar –** exfoliates the skin
- **Whole milk –** reduces acne, cleans and moisturizes. It is a well-known ingredient of the homemade remedies that women have used throughout the centuries. The biggest benefit is the fact that reduces skin pigmentation and gives a special brightness to the skin.
- **Eggs –** I know, we usually eat eggs. But why not try to benefit from all their vitamins and minerals by putting them on our face? The skin also needs vitamins and minerals. And the eggs can provide them: vitamin A, selenium, iodine, vitamin B12, B2, iron, calcium, phosphorus and potassium.

What You'll Need:

- ✓ 1 cup oat flakes
- ✓ 1 teaspoon sweet almond oil (or coconut/olive oil)
- ✓ 1 tablespoon brown sugar
- ✓ 1 egg white (or whole, it doesn't matter)
- ✓ 2 tablespoons whole milk

Directions:

1. Grind the oatmeal until you get a rough flour.

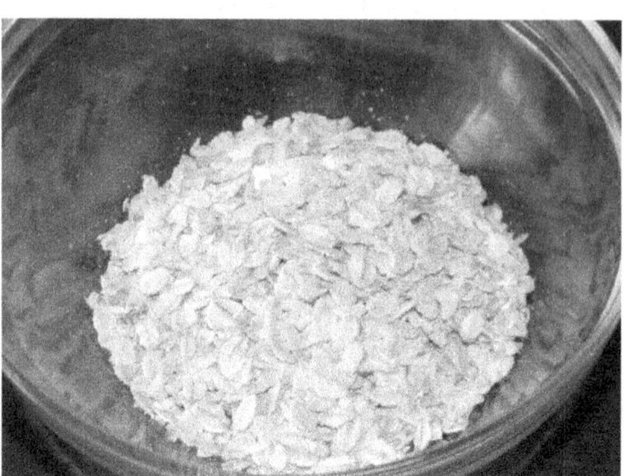
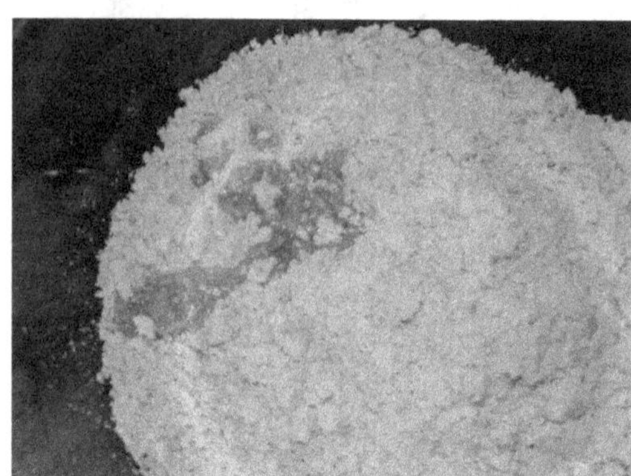

2. Combine all the ingredients in a bowl and mix them well. If you can't spread the mixture, add some more oil, few drops at a time.

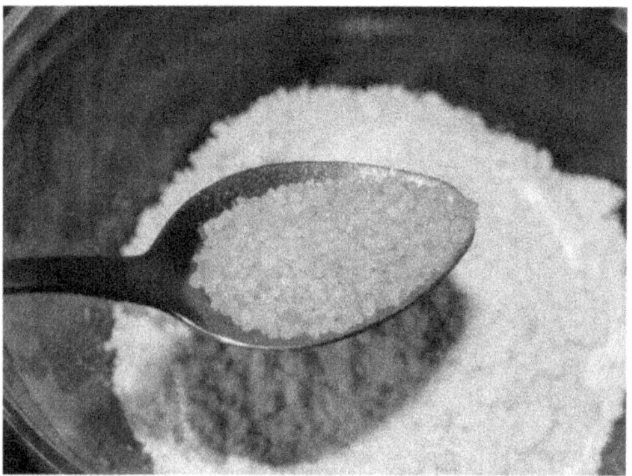
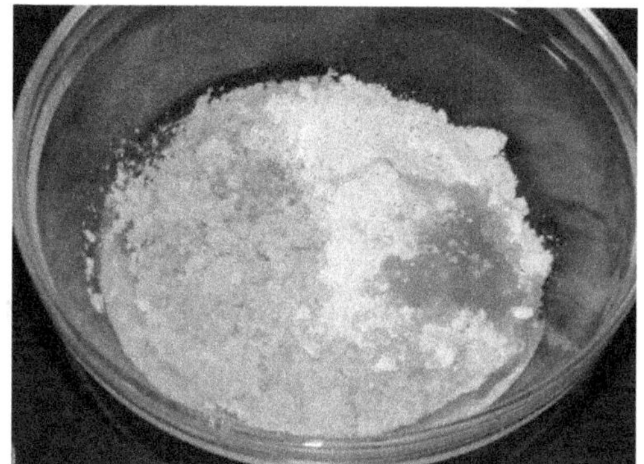

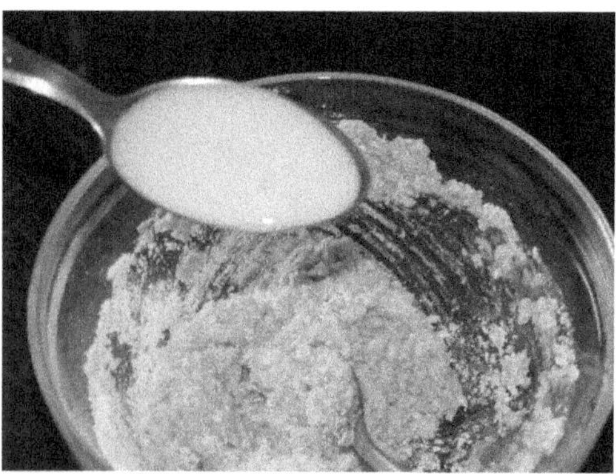
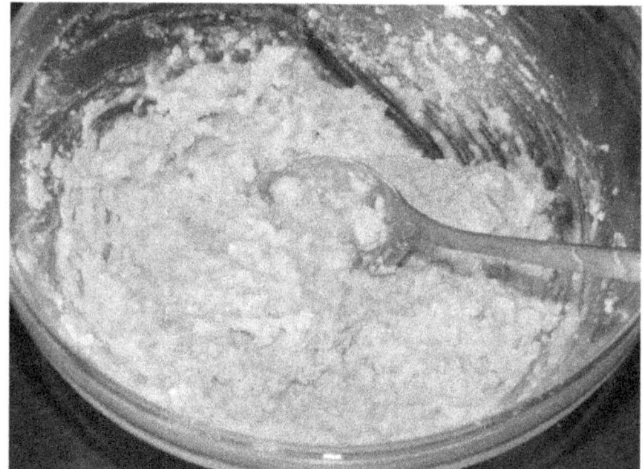

3. Apply the scrub with gentle moves on your face and neck.

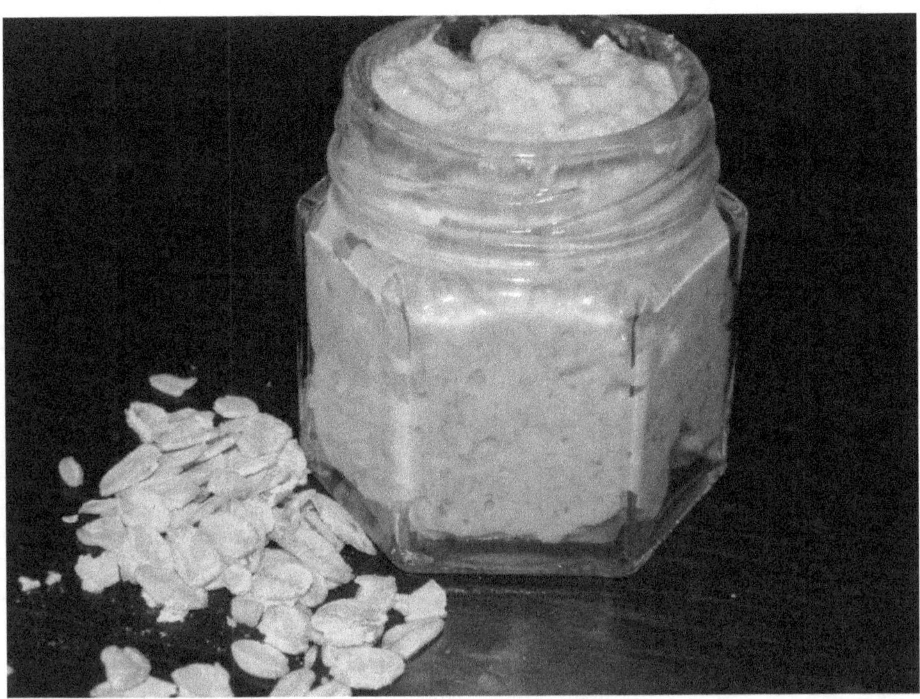

4. Rinse with warm water.

You should use this scrub at least once a week. Twice is best. I can promise you that your skin will glow, especially if you combine the scrub with a homemade face lotion.

Oil Cleansing Ritual

Have you ever thought that you could clean your face using natural oils? I must admit that I found it quite strange when I first heard of such thing. I have combined skin and I thought that an oil will make my face more oily, right?

Not quite so. There is a principle in chemistry: to solve the problems of oily skin it is advisable to use a substance similar in composition: another oil. The benefits of this cleansing ritual which uses natural oils are undeniable because the skin will not come into contact with the chemical ingredients found in traditional products.

First you will face a detoxifying process for the skin to get rid of all impurities trapped in pores over time. It is a short period, up to one week. It is possible that the skin seems loaded all this time because it eliminates toxins. But you must resist the urge to clean it with who knows what miracle chemical, hoping that things will work out. This will actually happen: your face will look much better after getting rid of all the impurities that clog pores. You only need a little patience :)

The good news is that this method works for any skin type. Using natural oils regulates the secretion of natural sebum, unlike conventional cleaning products that have the opposite effect and lead to an imbalance.

What You'll Need:

- ✓ Cold pressed olive oil
- ✓ Cold pressed castor oil (castor oil is a natural astringent that helps eliminate toxins from the skin)

Directions:

Depending on your skin type, you can combine the two oils as follows:

- **Oily Skin:** 1/3 parts castor oil and 2/3 parts olive oil
- **Combined Skin:** 1/4 parts castor oil and 3/4 parts olive oil
- **Dry Skin:** Olive oil and add very little castor oil

To find out the right combination for your skin, you should use small amounts to begin with, for example, 1 teaspoon of castor oil with 2 teaspoons of olive oil for oily skin. Adjust the amount depending on the way your skin feels.

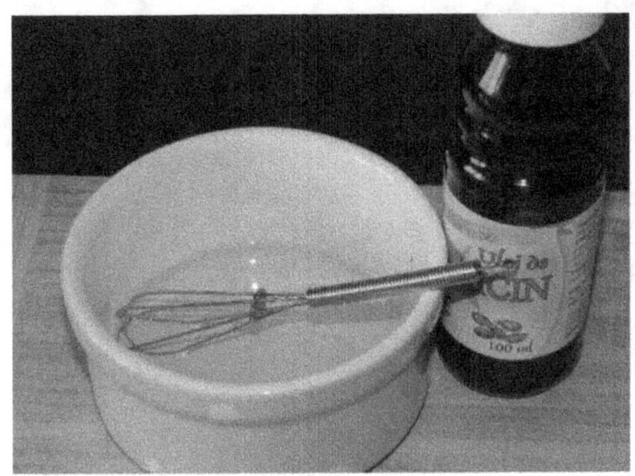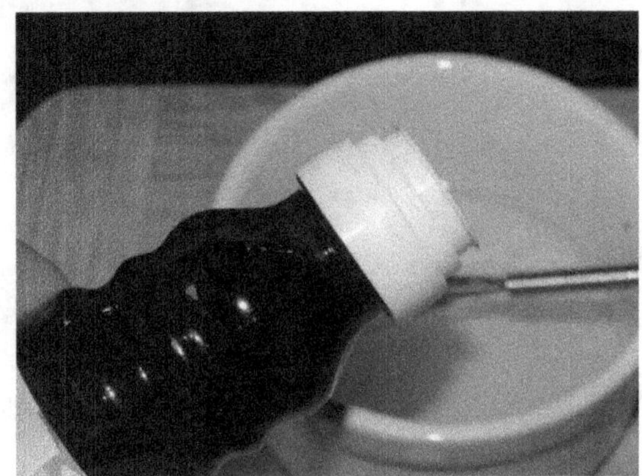

What To Do Next?

Gently massage the face with the oil mixture. Use circular movements so you don't irritate the skin. The massage should last 1-2 minutes. You can even leave the mixture on for 10 minutes or until you feel that your skin is moisturized. It is necessary for skin to be dry before you apply the oils. Makeup does not necessarily need to be removed, as the oils will handle this.

Soak a clean towel in hot water, squeeze it well and then cover your face with it. Steam will help the pores to open and eliminate impurities. Keep the towel on your face for a minute. Use the towel edges to wipe off any oil traces left.

Normally, it should not be necessary to apply a moisturizer after this process. If you do feel the need, try to reduce the amount of astringent oil used for the cleansing ritual and apply a natural lotion.

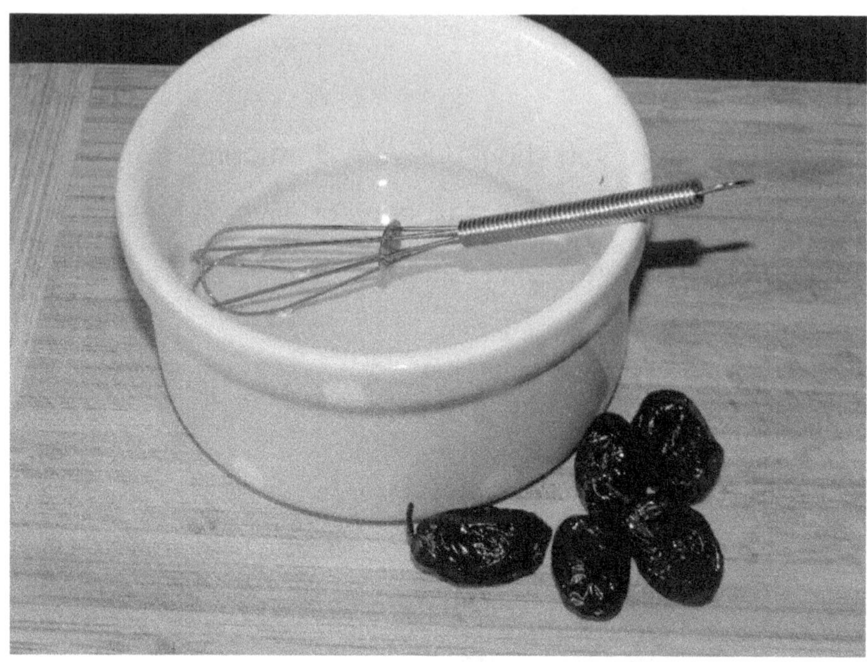

Olive Oil and Brown Sugar Scrub

I simply love preparing my own natural cosmetics. They are less expensive than the trade ones and I know exactly what ingredients I use. I especially like beauty recipes with few ingredients and easy to prepare. Like the face scrub below: only two ingredients and a lot of benefits.

As you know, brown sugar is excellent for exfoliating the skin and keep it healthy.

What About The Olive Oil?

- It is rich in vitamins and antioxidants and can be used for treating acne because it deeply cleanses the skin, removes impurities and leaves the epidermis glowing.
- Thanks to the antioxidants, olive oil is one of the main ingredient used in the preparation of anti-aging cosmetics.
- It is rich in protein, minerals, vitamins and essential fatty acids which are beneficial for dehydrated skin.
- Olive oil protects the skin from the harmful effects of free radicals, preventing skin aging.

Therefore, the mask containing olive oil and brown sugar will be able to successfully remove all the dead cells and leave your face young and shiny.

What You'll Need:

- ✓ 1 tablespoon brown sugar
- ✓ 1 teaspoon olive oil (you may adjust the oil quantity, by adding or removing few drops so you reach the desired consistency for this mask)

Directions:

1. You may use a small bowl to mix the two ingredients or just combine them on your palm.
2. First place the brown sugar.

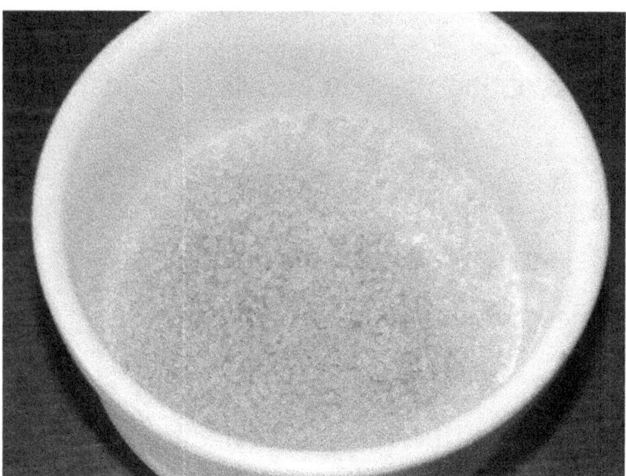

3. Slowly add the olive oil so that you form a paste.

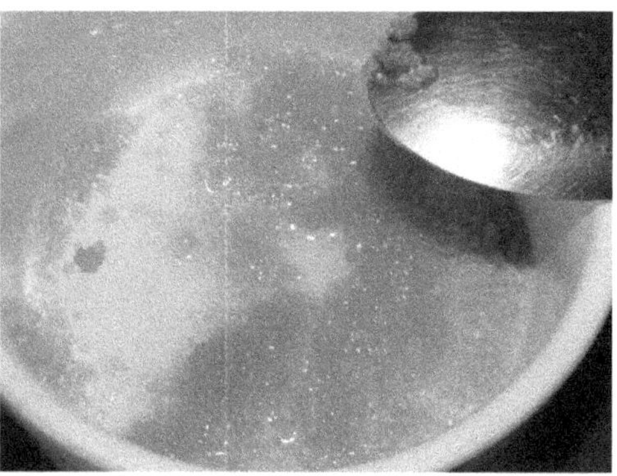 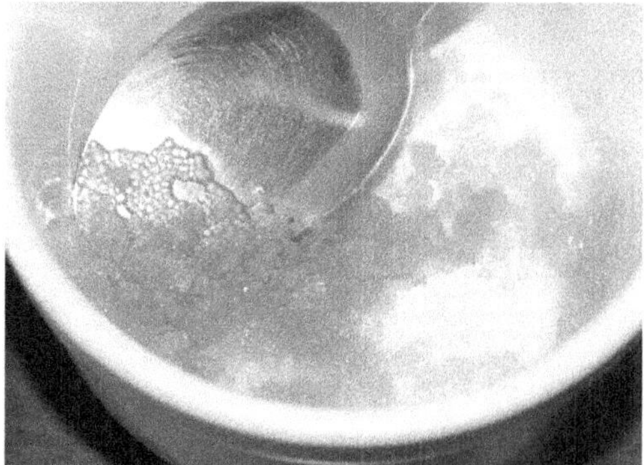

4. Apply the mixture to your face and neck, using circular, gentle moves.

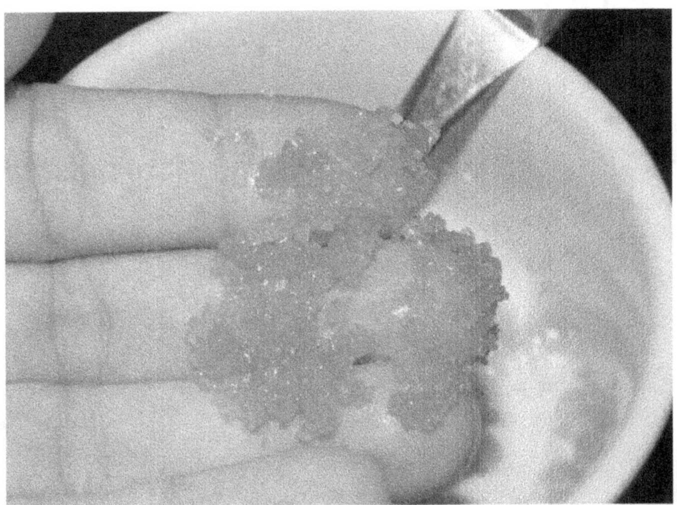

5. Massage the face so that you remove all the dead cells and allow the olive oil to moisturize the skin.
6. Rinse with warm water.
7. Wipe your face with a warm, soft towel.

If you wish to prepare a larger quantity of this scrub, simply multiply the quantities and keep it in a dry airtight container. Use whenever you have time to. A deep face cleansing is always welcome.

The classic cleanser is often irritating to the eyes. It is possible that you get some red, swollen eyes by using some chemicals to remove your make-up. So, why don't forget about those conventional cleansing lotions and try to prepare your own using only natural ingredients?

The eye cleanser from this recipe uses a combination of ingredients that are perfect for eye care.

What You'll Need:

- ✓ 1 tbsp castor oil
- ✓ 2 tbsp sweet almond oil
- ✓ 2 tbsp cornflower water

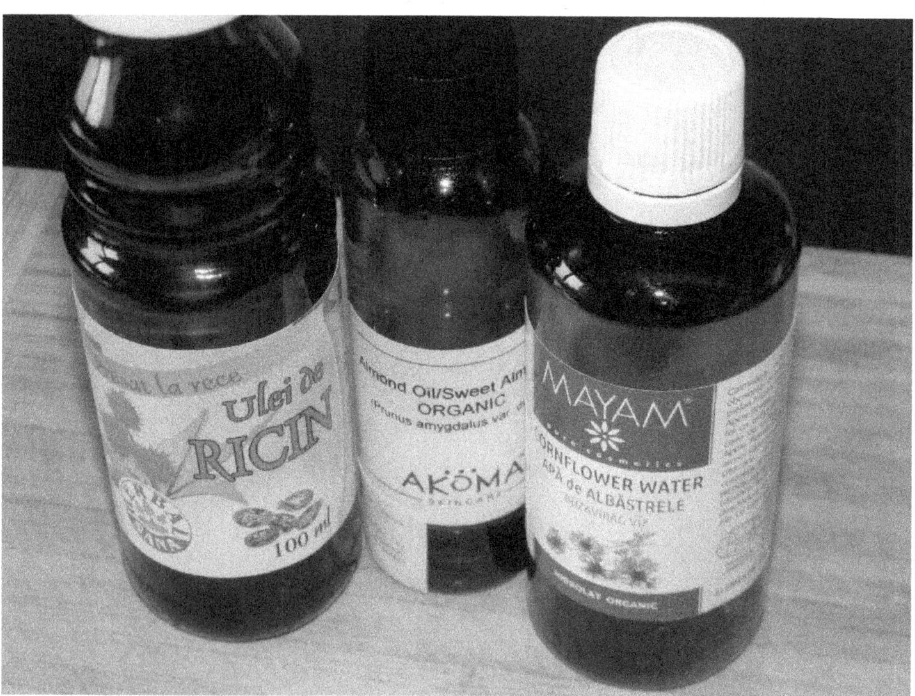

Directions:

1. Combine all the ingredients in a cup.

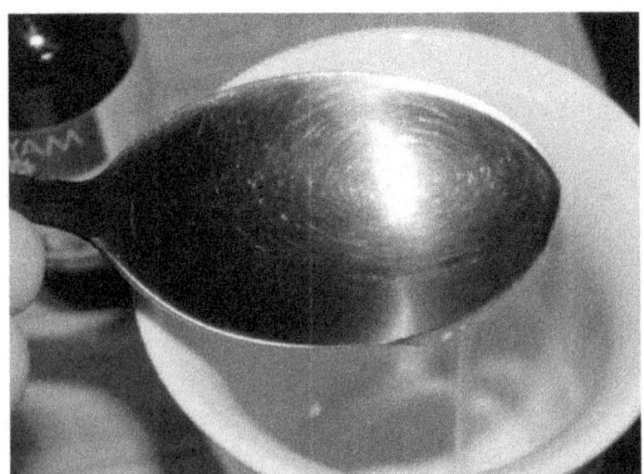 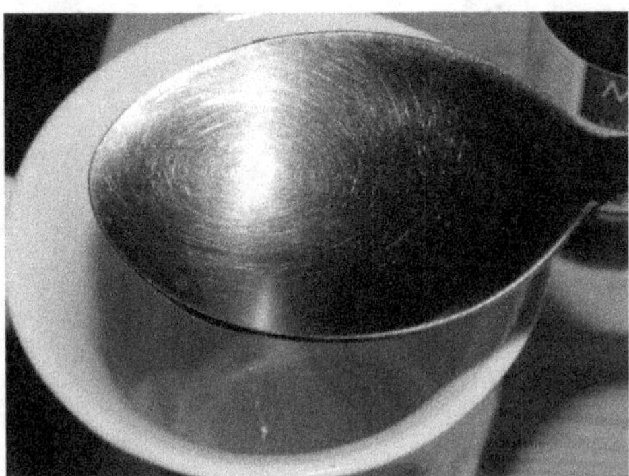

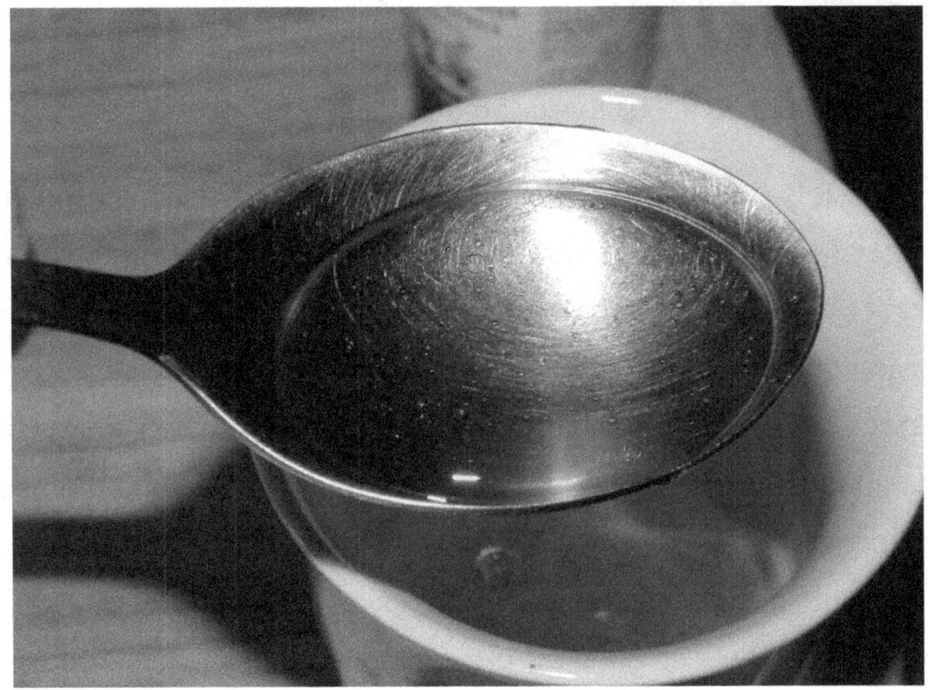

2. Mix all the ingredients together, then transfer them to a glass jar, put the lid on and shake well.

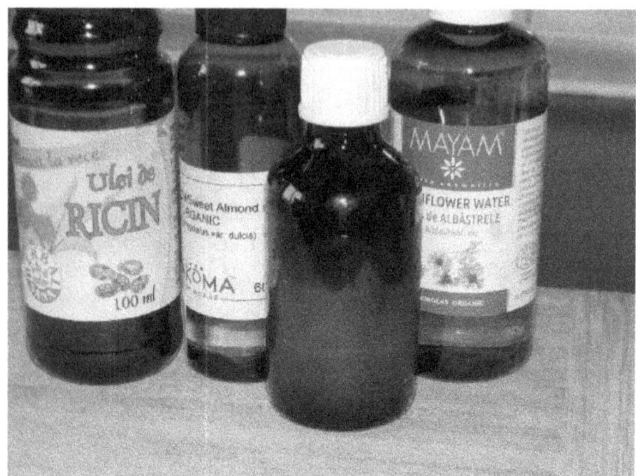

3. Keep the cleanser in the fridge for no more than 2 weeks.
4. Shake well before each use.

So, let me tell you something about these three ingredients:

- **Castor oil** – it is a natural derivative which, by its properties, is used in a wide range of cosmetic beauty treatments but also for prevention, control or correction of various body diseases. In addition to its antibacterial, anti-fungal and antiviral properties, castor oil contains a large number of antioxidants that help the body fight free radicals. It is also the only known source of unsaturated fatty acids and has a role in protecting the skin and the hair. The castor oil diminishes the dark areas under the eyes but also the wrinkles and keeps the skin's smoothness.
- **Sweet almond oil** – also good for preventing the dark circles. Nourishes the skin, making it smooth and soft. Soothes dry and itching skin. Almond oil can be used for the delicate skin under the eyes to prevent wrinkles.

- **Cornflower water** – Cornflower have anti-inflammatory, antiseptic, bacteriostatic, emollient and soothing properties. In case of eye problems, cornflower water can be used for eyewash or compresses to the eyelids. Compresses with cornflower water are recommended especially for wrinkles on the eyelids or tired and irritated eyes. Due to soothing and toning effect cornflower treatments are recommended for facial muscles and wrinkles.

I simply adore strawberries. My kids do too. We eat tones of them. We can't seem to stop eating. Lucky my husband comes in and takes the bowl out of our face. We could probably spend an entire day eating strawberries :)

Recently I have found out that they are not only delicious, but very healthy too. And good for the skin. So I've decided to prepare a strawberry scrub for my face.

I had a few reasons for doing that:

- One of the many wonders of strawberries is the salicylic acid they contain. It has the effect of removing dead cells, reduces pores and makes the skin brighter.
- Very rich in vitamins and minerals (vitamin C, potassium, iron, sodium), strawberries exfoliate, remove impurities, and also reduce redness and swelling stains. Antioxidants from strawberries repair the skin by stimulating the production of new cells. Hence the next big benefit of these fruits: anti-aging effect.
- Strawberries are recommended for people with oily skin because of their astringent properties. These fruits improve skin texture and reduce the sebum oil in excess. But if you want to refresh your skin, you can use a strawberry mask if you have dry or normal skin as well.

What You'll Need:

- ✓ 2 tablespoons brown sugar
- ✓ 1 tablespoon sweet almond oil
- ✓ 2 strawberries

Directions:

1. Chop the strawberries in very small pieces or smash them.

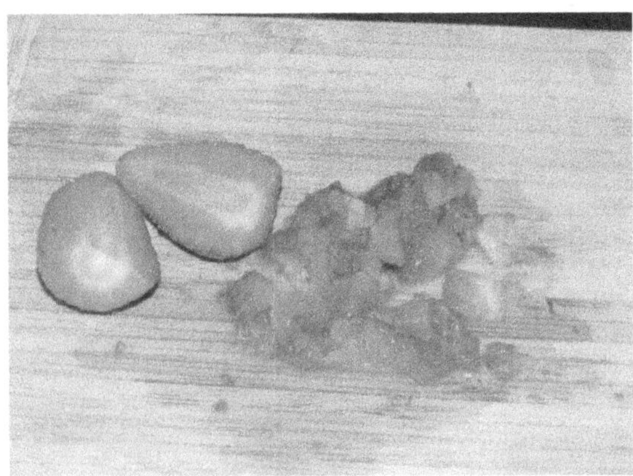

2. Combine the brown sugar and the sweet almond oil.

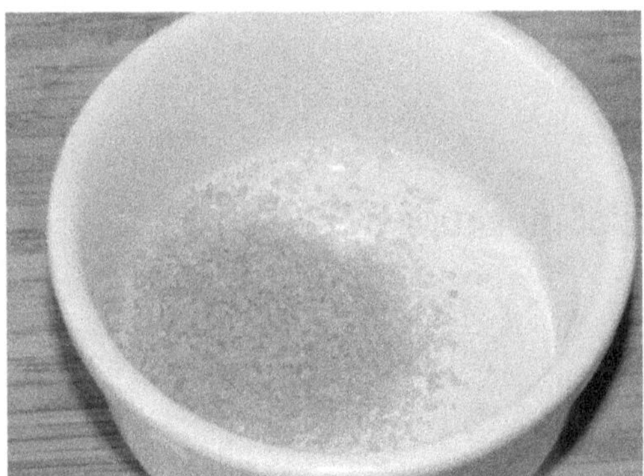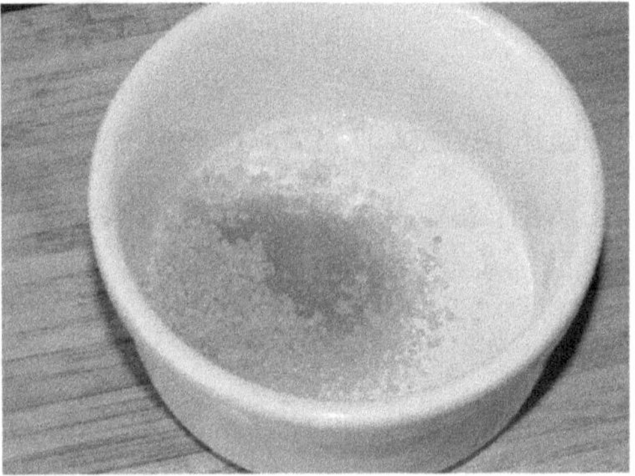

3. Add the strawberries to the mixture and stir well.

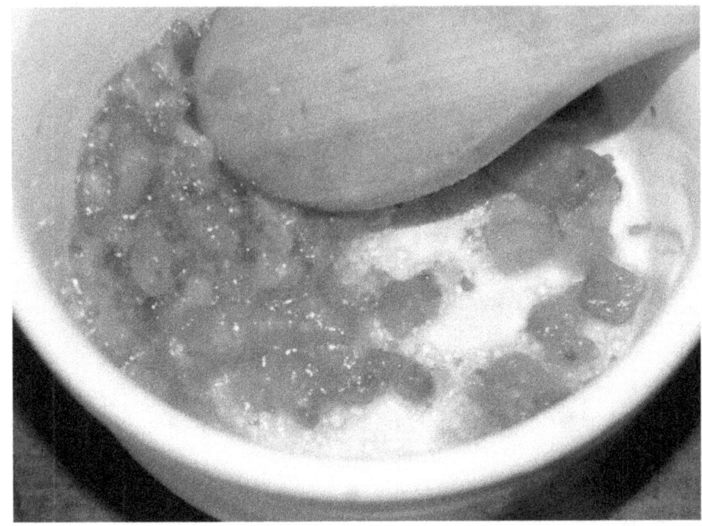

4. Apply the scrub on the face and neck with soft, circular moves. Massage gently for 3-5 minutes and let the salicylic acid take action.

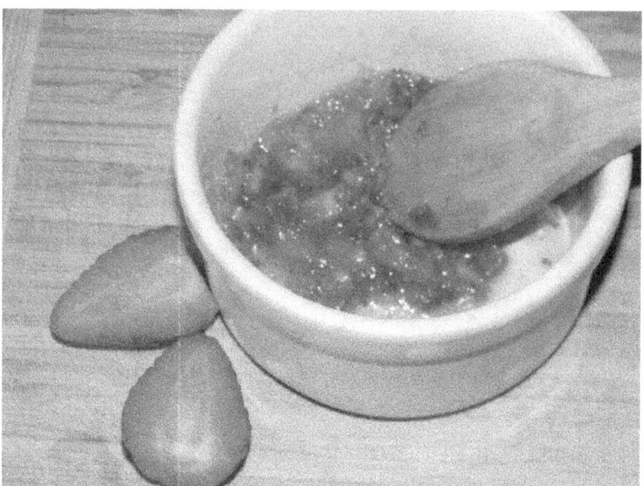

5. Wash your face with warm water.
6. Wipe it with a warm towel, then apply a facial moisturizer.

I believe it's amazing that you can put some food on your face and get a shiny, glowing skin. Let me tell you some things about tomatoes and their benefits for your skin.

Tomato masks are very useful for spots that appear due to direct exposure to the sunlight. They are also effective for those who have trouble with oily skin, acne or enlarged pores.

Tomatoes have so many benefits for the skin because of their powerful nutrients like lycopene, protein, vitamin A and vitamin C. Lycopene, an antioxidant that gives the red color, fights free radicals in the body, which makes it a formidable weapon in treating skin problems.

There are other nutrients found in tomatoes which are considered a great help in solving skin problems: vitamin C and vitamin A make the dull skin shine and restore its health. Tomato also has astringent properties which means it removes excess sebum.

If all those sound good to you, try to use a tomato scrub at least once a week.

What You'll Need:

- ✓ 1 tablespoon olive oil
- ✓ 2 tablespoons sea salt
- ✓ ½ tomato

Directions:

1. Combine the sea salt and olive oil.

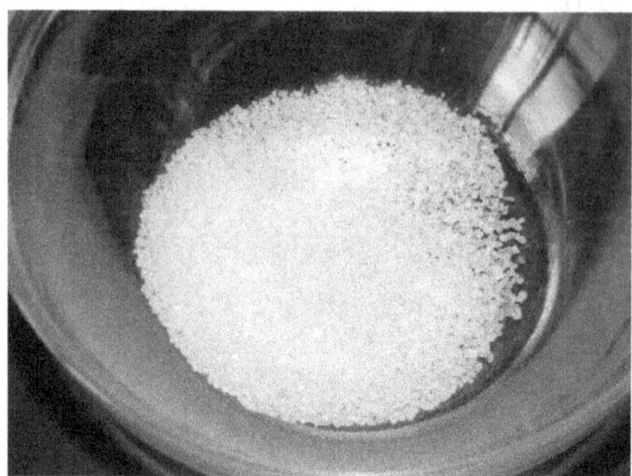 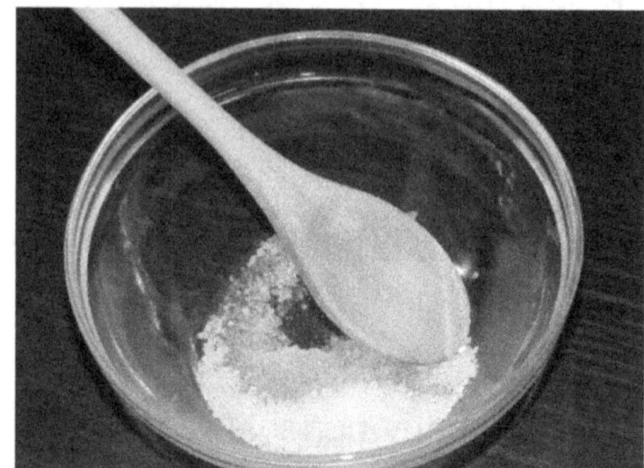

2. Mix in the tomato flesh.

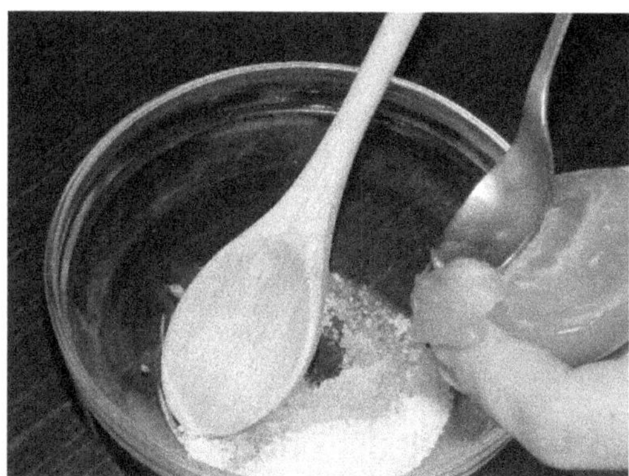 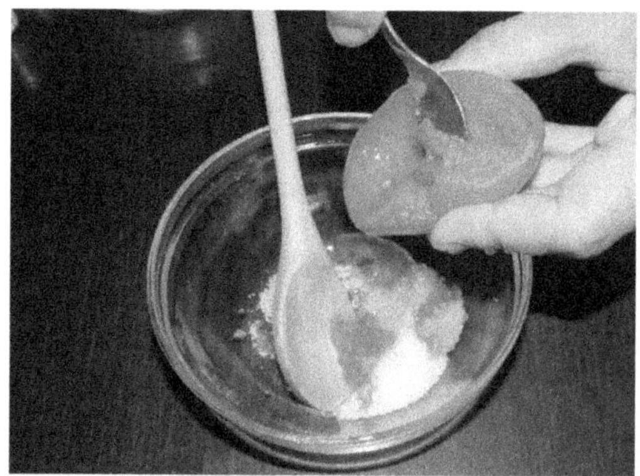

3. Stir well.

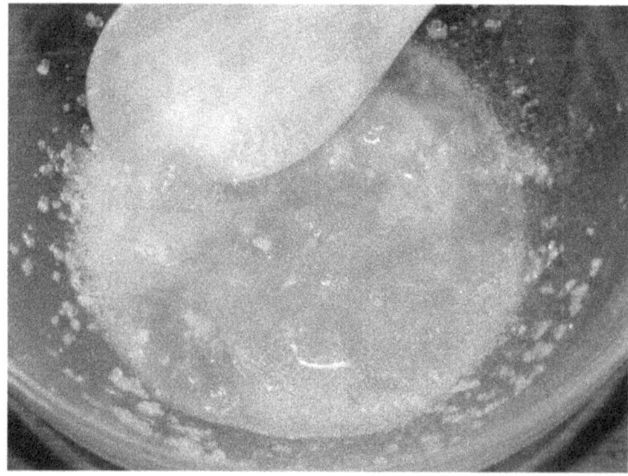 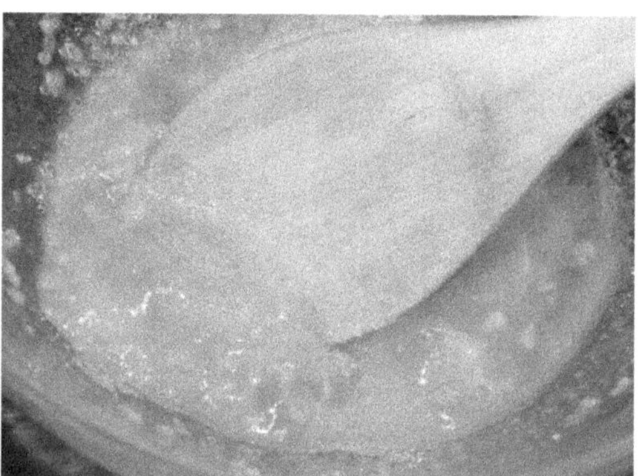

4. Apply to your face by gently massaging it.

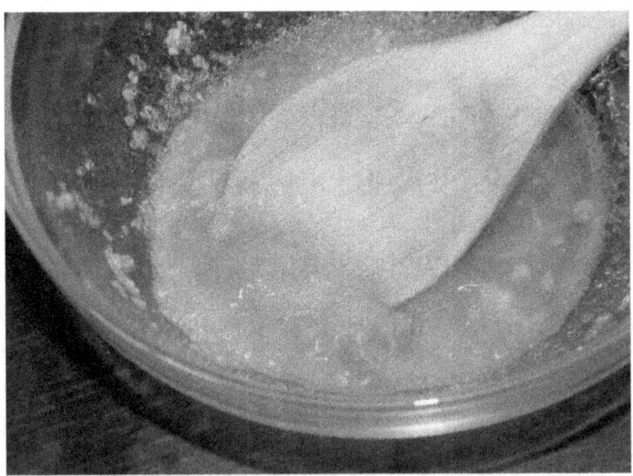

5. Rinse with warm water and apply your favorite moisturizer.
6. If you want to make a larger quantity of scrub, simply store it in a container. You can keep it in the fridge for up to 2 weeks.

Here's what this scrub can do for you:

- Efficiently cleans pores, removing dead cells and dirt from the face. Also, tomato juice reduces enlarged pores, acting as a natural astringent.
- Removes blackheads, moisturizes oily skin and reduces the oily appearance. Tomatoes are recommended for treating irritations and redness by balancing the pH levels.
- Reduces acne. Although the results appear in time, applying a tomato mask helps cure acne. The skin will be more supple as tomatoes stimulate the production of collagen.

Yogurt is one of the most important nutritional foods to the body. Recently it has been proved to be beneficial for skin care as well.

Mostly everyone knows the benefits of yogurt consumption. It is very good for the immune system and at the same time, the best natural food for digestion.

Thanks to its high content in living bacteria which is beneficial to the body, yogurt can be applied to the skin too, not only ingested. In addition, many types of yogurt contain probiotics, some living micro-organisms that help maintain a balanced and healthy digestive system. Many studies have shown that women who eat yogurt are less prone to infection.

Also active substances in yogurt reduce the risk of colon cancer, decrease high blood pressure and prevent osteoporosis.

Yogurt can be applied to the skin for cleaning and moisturizing. It can be used on any skin type. Being rich in lactic acid, it is beneficial for mature skin as well.

So, we can use yogurt and eggs to prepare a hydrating and cleansing mask, rated by model Shalom Harlow as "moisturizing and soothing".

Eggs are also good for the skin as they bring an important intake of protein, minerals and vitamins.

What You'll Need:

- ✓ 2 tablespoons of plain yogurt
- ✓ 2 egg whites

Directions:

1. First of all, separate the egg whites.

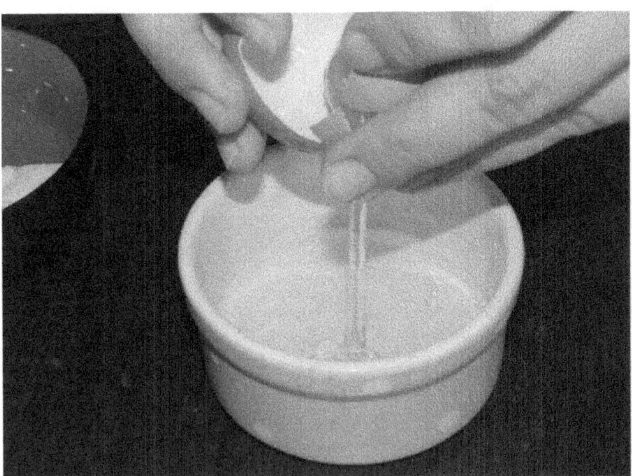

2. Whisk them in a bowl.
3. Add two tablespoons of yogurt (plain, not flavored) and mix well.

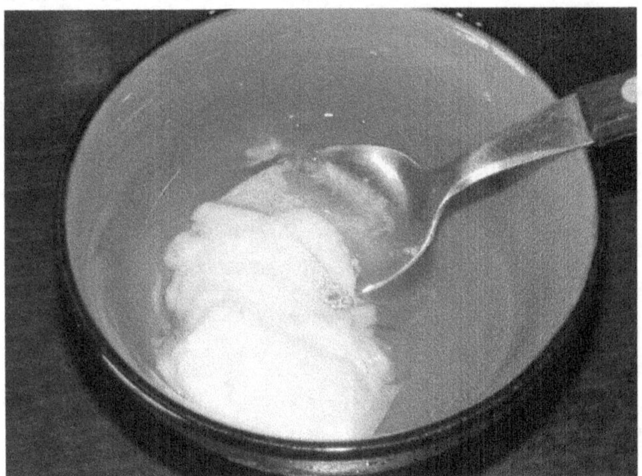

4. Apply this mixture on the face with gentle moves.

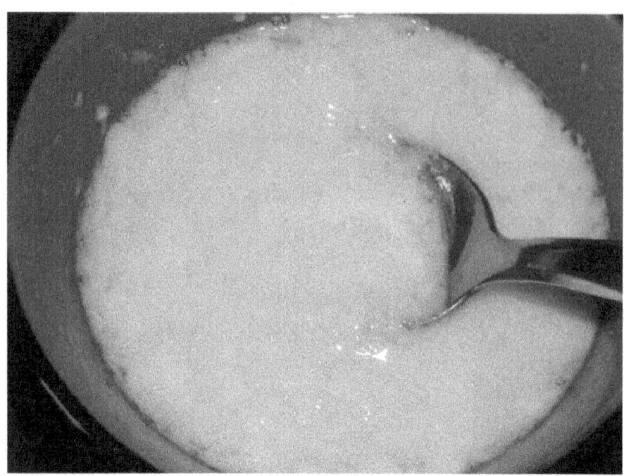

5. Leave it there for at least 5 minutes.
6. Use warm water to rinse the mask.
7. Wipe the face with a warm towel.

I enjoy this particular mask as it is super easy to make. Just open the fridge, take a look inside and get the yogurt and eggs. What can be more wonderful than to keep your skin healthy and shiny with food? Both eaten or put on your face. I am positive that our great grandmothers also used this kind of treatments as they didn't have innovative anti-aging serums to buy.

Yogurt Cleansing Lotion

The best cleansing lotions are the ones made with ingredients from your kitchen. They are not expensive but very efficient and healthy, as well.

And we must think about our grandmothers and their grandmothers which didn't have any fancy lotions to take care of their faces and used only stuff from their kitchens to put on their skin.

What You'll Need:

- ✓ 8 oz filtered or boiled water
- ✓ 1 oz whole yogurt
- ✓ 1/2 tsp dried calendula flowers (ground)
- ✓ 1/2 tsp dried thyme (ground)

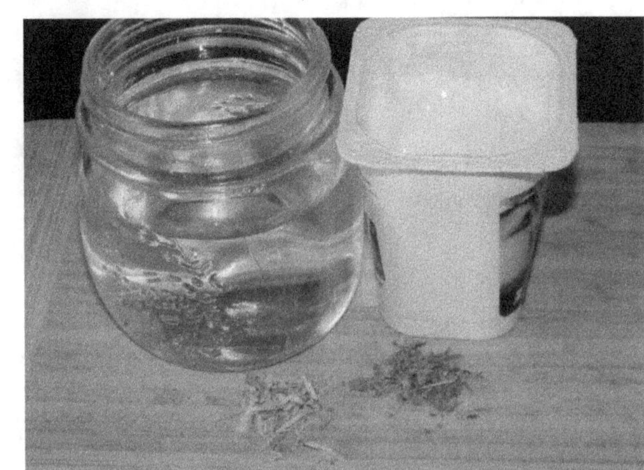

Directions:

1. Combine all the ingredients in a glass jar.

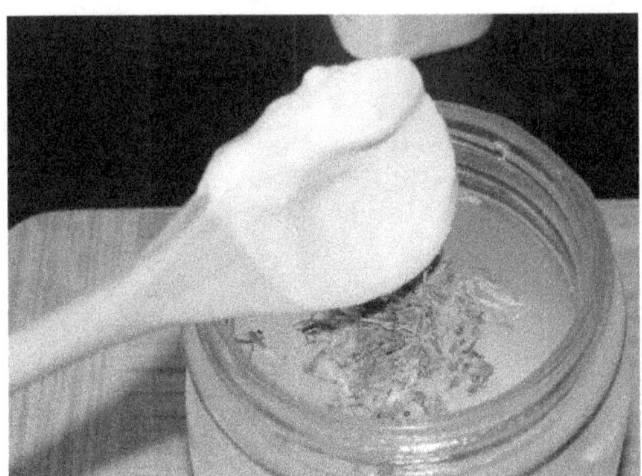
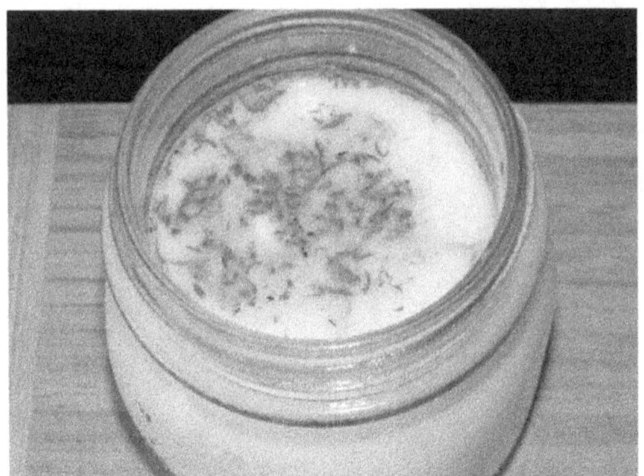

2. Put the lid on and let it in the fridge for 24 hours.

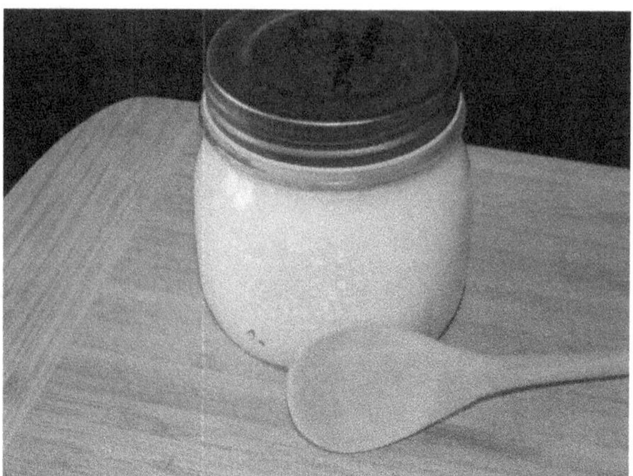

3. Take it out and blend the mixture. You face cleansing lotion is ready.
4. Place some mixture on a cotton pad and cleanse you face using gentle moves until it is smooth and soft.
5. Rinse any residue with warm water.
6. Apply your favorite moisturizer.

Anti-Wrinkle, All-Natural Moisturizers

Beautiful, youthful skin is something that we all strive for. However, in our quest to look younger, we often use conventional skin care products which promise to smooth our skin and fight the visible signs of aging.

While these products may improve the appearance of our skin on an exterior level, they are extremely dangerous and loaded with harmful chemicals. These chemicals have a range of unpleasant side effects. They can irritate the skin and even interfere with the body's endocrine system.

So, how can you get smooth, young looking skin without using these products?

Anti-Wrinkle, All-Natural Moisturizers

All in One Face Cream

I use this cream for my face, but it can also be used for hands, body, feet, etc. It is extremely moisturizing, and it spreads easily. Although it may seem a little bit oily, the skin (mine, at least) absorbs it in about 10 minutes. I recommend you first try it at night, before you go to bed. I suppose you wouldn't like to have a greasy face on your way to work.

But I really doubt this could happen as natural oils are usually well absorbed by the skin as they have the capacity to dissolve the excess oils that stuck together with other impurities on our epidermis.

The ingredients from this lotion are all-natural and have a moisturizing and nourishing effect on your skin. It is always better to use a homemade face cream than a trade one. This way you can get rid of all the chemicals and parabens from the conventional cosmetic products.

I found the activity of creating my own lotions quite addictive. I'm sure you will too after you start it.

And what better moment to start than now, with this recipe?

You will need:

- ✓ 2 tbsp cocoa butter
- ✓ 2 tbsp shea butter
- ✓ 1 tbsp vegetable glycerin
- ✓ 20 drops Vitamin E oil
- ✓ 4 tbsp extra virgin olive oil
- ✓ 10 drops essential oil (you may use your favorite, I used 8 drops Lavender and 2 drops

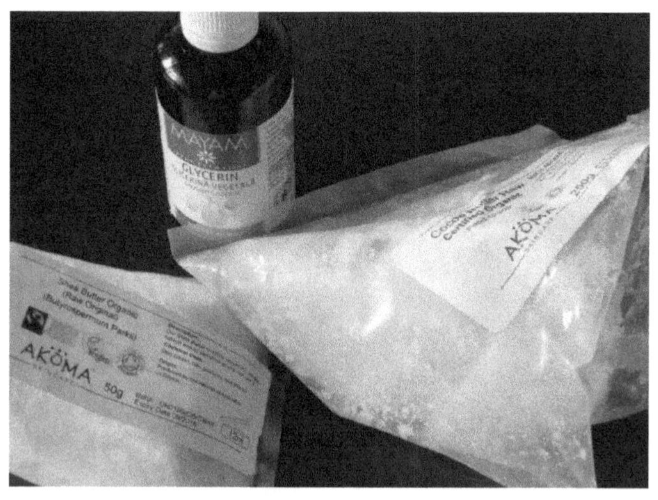

Peppermint)

Directions:

1. Mix together the cocoa and shea butter and the olive oil in a glass jar. I don't have a double boiler, so I put the jar in a small pan half filled with water. So, place the pan on low heat so that the butters melt.

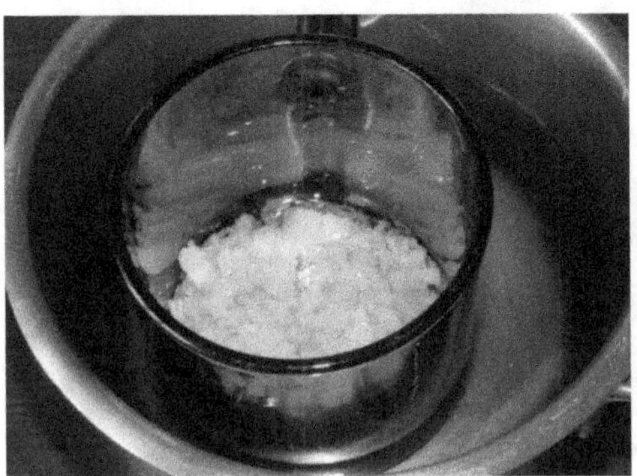
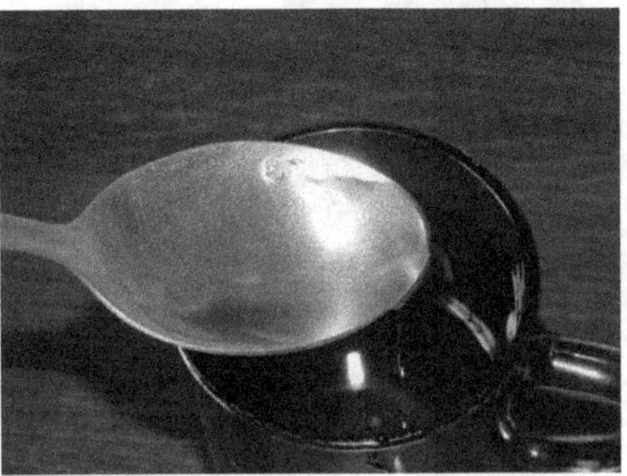

2. After that, remove from heat and add all the other ingredients.

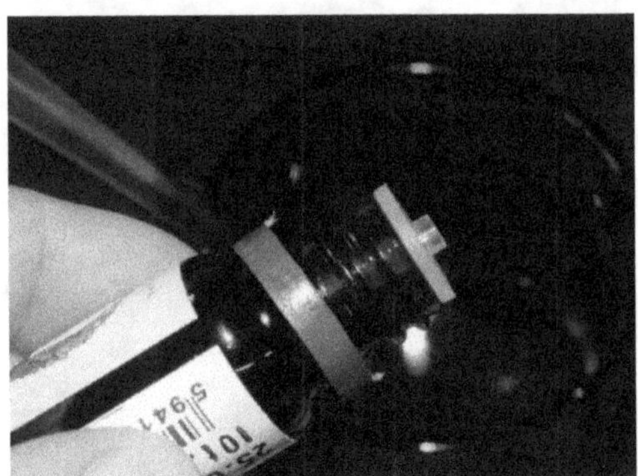
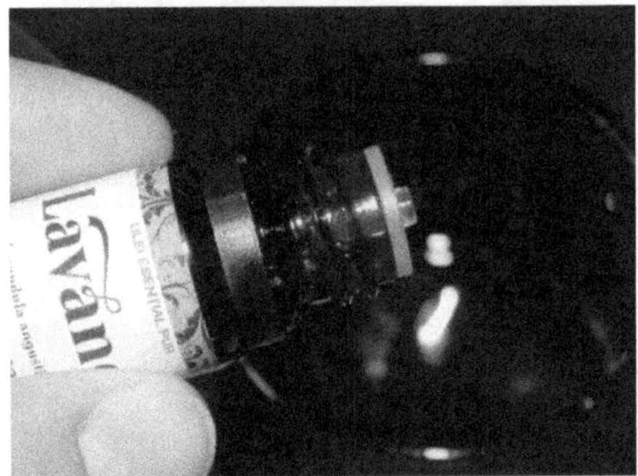

3. The mixture will cool completely after 12-24 hours.

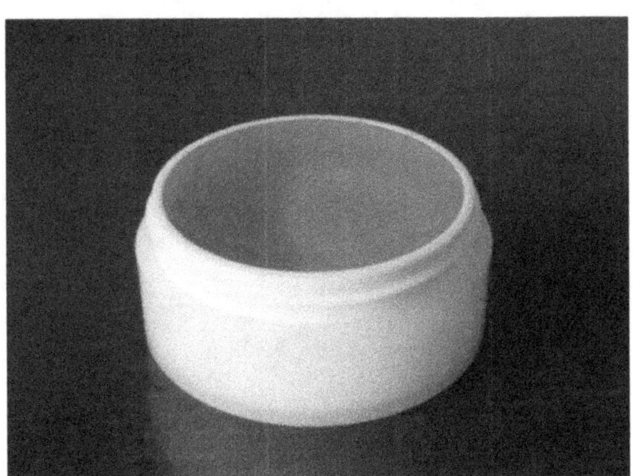

4. If you want a fluffy consistency, you may place it in the freezer after you remove it from heat.
5. Let it start to solidify again and whip it with a hand mixer.
6. You may store it at room temperature as it will not melt unless it is very hot.

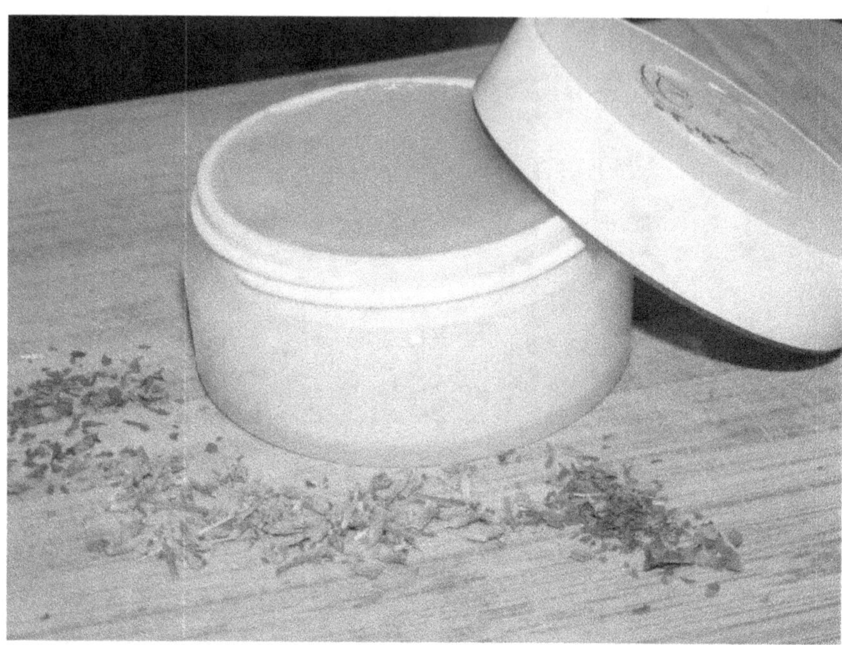

Aloe Vera Face Moisturizer

Did you know that aloe vera can cure almost all skin conditions, from severe dryness and premature aging to strong inflammation and burns caused by direct exposure to sun light?

Nicknamed "the miracle herb" or "natural medicine", aloe vera has been used for its therapeutic qualities for more than 4,000 years. Researchers show that a plant named aloe vera was used by the Egyptians, Greeks, Chinese and Indians to cure certain diseases, but also to adorn the body.

Today, aloe vera is a key ingredient for most cosmetics, because it comprises compounds that restore skin miraculously.

For example, the aloe plant contains more than 200 compounds, such as vitamins, minerals, amino acids, enzymes, polysaccharides, fatty acids, salicylic acid, antioxidants, flavonoids. In translation, this means that aloe contains all the important nutrients that our body needs. Over time, aloe vera has undergone countless research. There were conducted over 200 studies on this plant, research including three major categories of properties: anti-inflammatory, antibacterial and antiviral.

The healing range of the aloe vera plant is widespread, the juice of the plant is used for sunburn, eczema, psoriasis, acne, bruises, cuts, and the list goes on.

So, we should use it in our homemade lotions, right?

You will need:

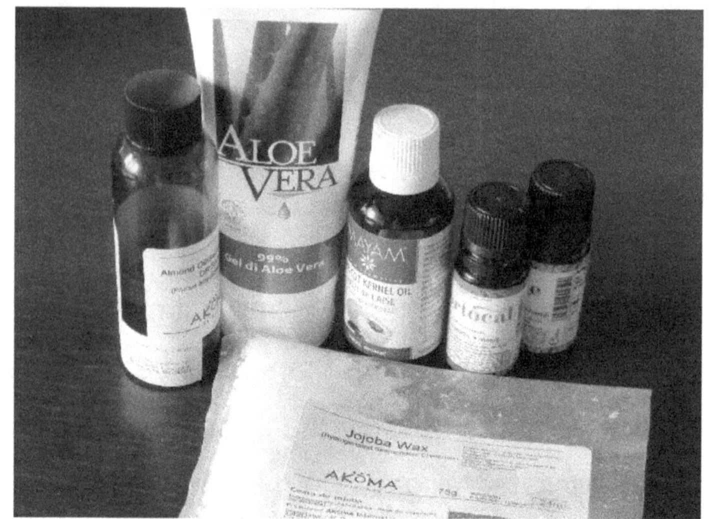

- 2 tbsp sweet almond oil
- 1/3 cup aloe vera gel
- 2 tbsp apricot kernel oil
- 1 tbsp jojoba wax/beeswax (I used jojoba)
- 10 drops essential oil (I used orange and lemon)

Directions:

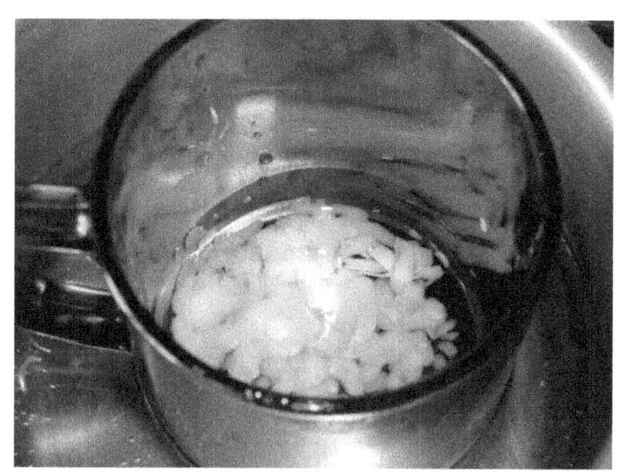

1. Combine all the oils (except for the essential ones) in a glass bowl. Place it in a pan half filled with water.
2. Let it over low heat until the wax melts.
3. Remove from heat and let it cool until it gets to room temperature.
4. Add the essential oils to the aloe vera gel.
5. Slowly pour the gel to the oil mixture using a hand mixer.
6. Whip until it gets a butter consistency.

Enjoy!

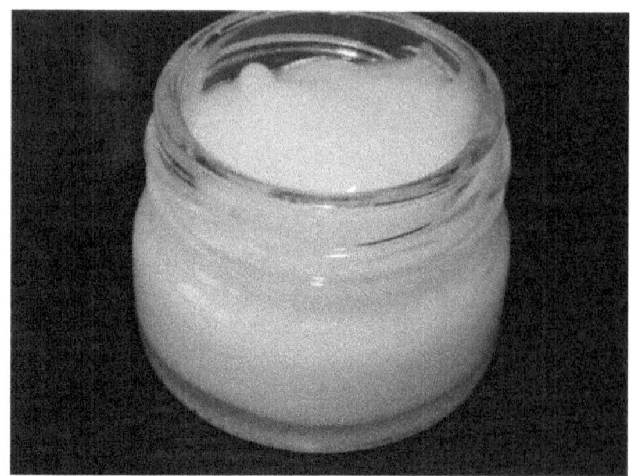

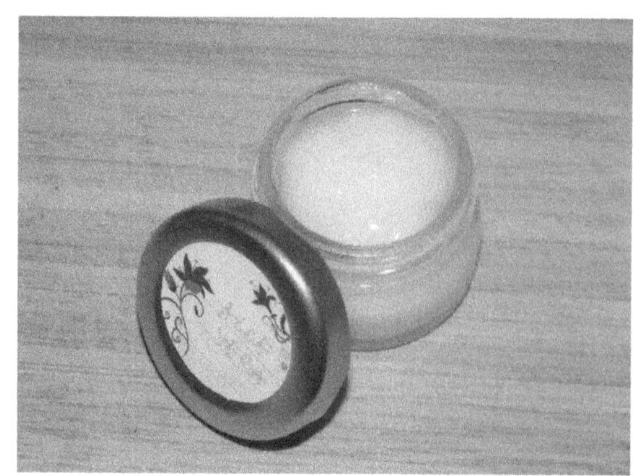

GE 55

Argan Oil Face Cream

Did I ever mention that between me and argan oil was love at first sight/use? I simply adore its soft texture, its nutty smell and the way my face feels after I apply it.

It is said that any moisturizer is good for preventing wrinkles as they appear faster on dry skin. So, besides the fact that it is an excellent hydrating oil, what else makes argan oil to be so effective against wrinkles (compared to other oils or creams)? When you see a bottle of argan oil, you should notice, in fact, a bottle full of antioxidants: vitamin E, vitamin A, unsaturated fatty acids. All these components have been studied and has been shown they that can prevent wrinkles and other health problems.

It has a light texture and is absorbed quickly, so there are no greasy traces after using it. It has no side effects, and the skin does not dry out when no longer in use. It regenerates skin during sleep and fight against skin aging. Being very rich in unsaturated fatty acids and containing a large amount of linoleic acid, argan oil is a good correction of the deficiencies of fatty acids in the skin, so important in delaying aging.

If you want to enter the pure argan oil in daily moisturizing ritual, you should know that 2 drops are enough for face and neck. Massage with gentle movements to take full advantage of all the nutrients.

After few months of using only argan oil for my face, I've decided to try to combine it with some other ingredients and to prepare a face cream and I used the below recipe.

You will need:

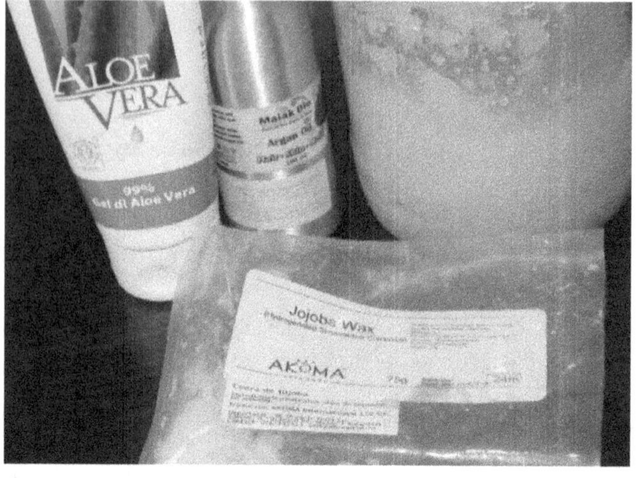

- 1 tsp sweet almond oil
- ½ tsp raw honey
- ½ tsp jojoba wax
- 1 ½ tsp aloe vera gel
- 5 drops argan oil

Directions:

1. Pour water into a small pan and place it over low heat.
2. Transfer the wax into a small jar and put it in the pan.
3. Let it melt and add the almond oil and the honey.
4. When everything is liquid, remove from heat.
5. Slowly mix in the aloe vera gel and the argan oil.
6. Stir until everything is well combined.
7. Pour the mixture into a glass container and let it cool.
8. Use as a day or night cream.

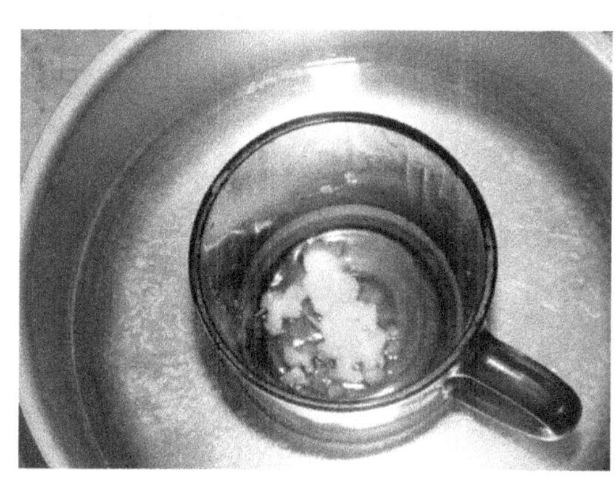

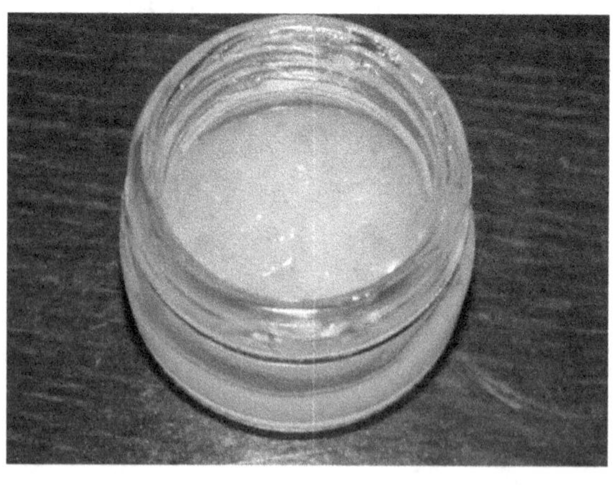

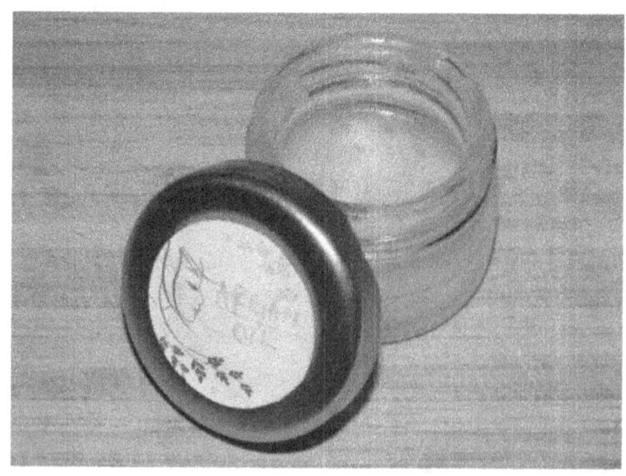

Facial Moisturizer for Dry Skin

My mom has had a dry face since forever. All her life she's tried to find a moisturizer that would make her skin soft. Some of them seemed to work, but most of them didn't. She also tried natural oils and butters and used them as they were, not combined. But she wasn't happy with them either.

Lately, I've discovered a facial moisturizer recipe for dry skin. I made it and gave it to my mother to try it. She told me that for the first time in her life she felt her face hydrated. I was so happy to hear this that I promised I will prepare this moisturizer for ever and ever :)

It is not hard to make, it contains only natural ingredients and I believe that it's the oil combination that makes it so good for the dry skin.

If you suffer from the same ailment, I strongly suggest that you try it. It is a lot cheaper than the luxury lotions you may find in cosmetic stores that promise the whole world to you and usually don't deliver it.

You will need:

- 3 tbsp apricot kernel oil
- 3 tbsp avocado oil
- 3 tbsp sweet almond oil
- 3 tbsp rosewater
- 3 tbsp jojoba/beeswax

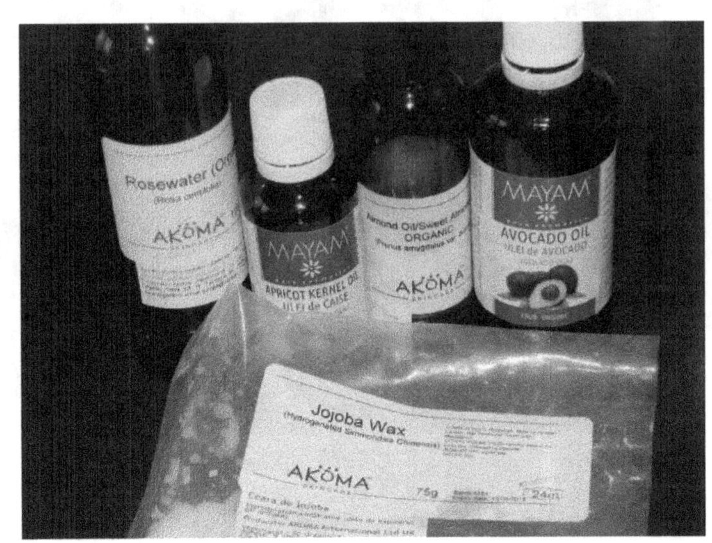

Directions:

1. Place the oil and the wax in a jar.
2. Put the jar in pan half filled with water over low heat.
3. Stir until the wax is melt and everything is well incorporated.
4. Remove the jar from the heat and let it cool a little bit by stirring continuously.
5. Slowly mix in the rose water.
6. Keep stirring until the mixture becomes smooth and it is completely cold.
7. Store in a dry container.
8. Keep it in the fridge or in a dark, cool place.
9. Use as a facial moisturizer whenever you need it.

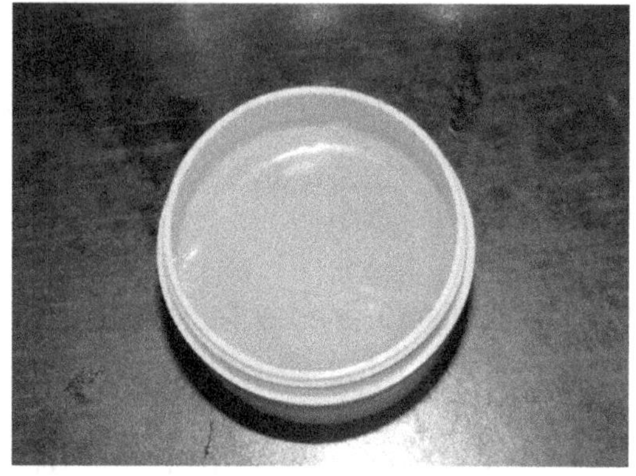

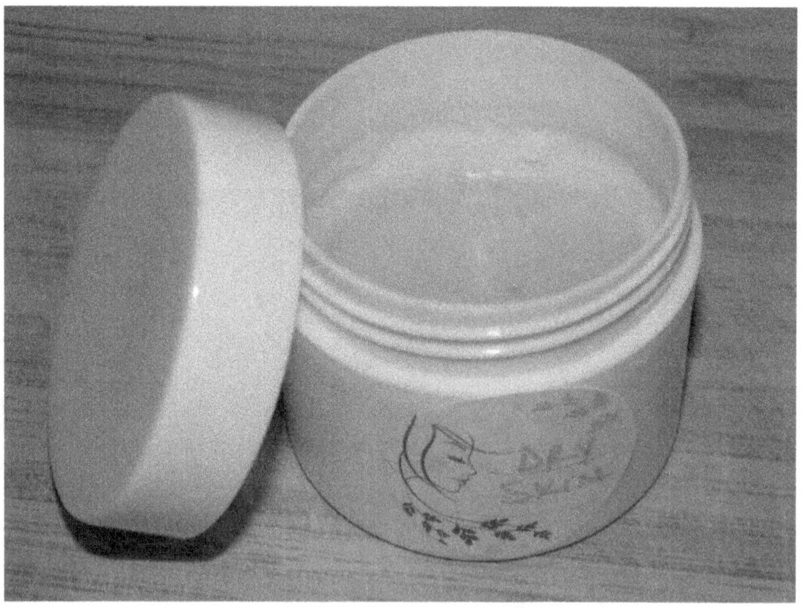

Facial Moisturizer for Normal Skin

All my life I had to take care of my oily skin. After I began to use only natural (organic or homemade) lotions for my face, my skin regained its oil balance. It looks amazing and I don't have to worry for grease traces or shining face anymore.

This is the reason I am using a moisturizer for normal skin now. It is also made with only natural ingredients and its role is to hydrate and keep the skin toned and healthy.

If you start using these homemade lotions, you will see how the quality of your epidermis is improving every day. Besides preparing them (which, from my point of view, is an extremely relaxing and pleasant activity), the only thing you need to do is to remember using them.

I believe I'm not the only one who used to buy a lot of lotions and face creams which expired in my cupboard, either because I was disappointed in them and didn't want to place them on my face anymore or because I simply forgot to use them. And, from time to time, I just removed them from the shelf when their life was gone.

The thing with homemade lotions is that I make them with my own hands. And I am so proud of the final result that I just know in my heart that I have to use all of it, until the last drop :)

So, for the facial moisturizer for normal skin, you will need:

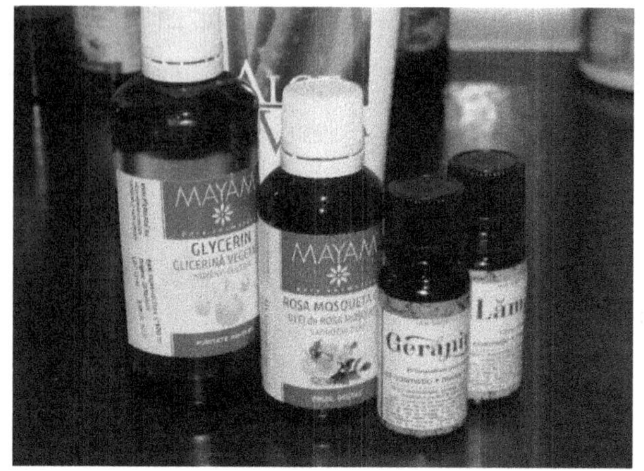

- 2 tbsp aloe vera gel
- 1 tsp dried herbs (I used calendula and chamomile)
- about 1 oz hot water
- 2 tbsp jojoba wax/beeswax
- ½ tsp vegetable glycerin
- 3 drops Rosa Mosqueta oil
- 6 drops of your favorite essential oil (I used Geranium and Lemon)

Directions:

1. Add the dried herbs to a glass bowl.

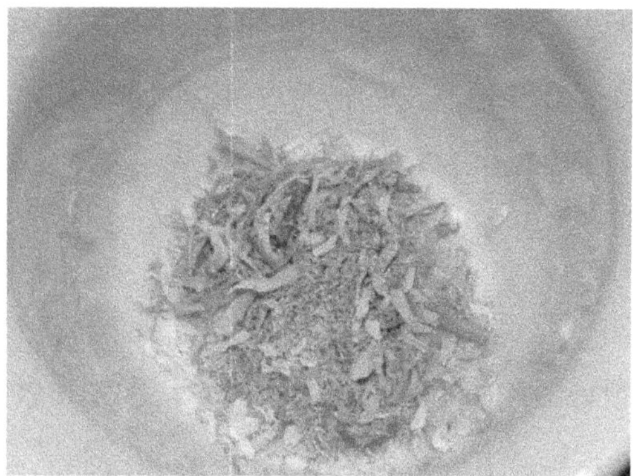

2. Pour the hot water over the dried herbs and let steep for at least 10 minutes.

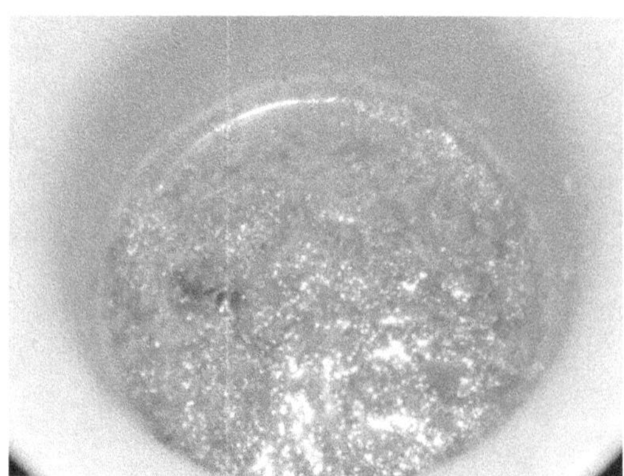

3. Drain the liquid and put it aside.

4. Combine the wax with the oils (except for the essential ones).

5. Pour some water into a pan and put the jar in.

6. Place the pan over low heat and melt the wax.

7. Remove the jar from heat and begin stirring until it gets colder.

8. Mix in slowly the plant liquid, the glycerin and the aloe vera gel until you get the desired consistency.

9. Store it in a dry container.

10. Keep it in the fridge or a dark, cool place.

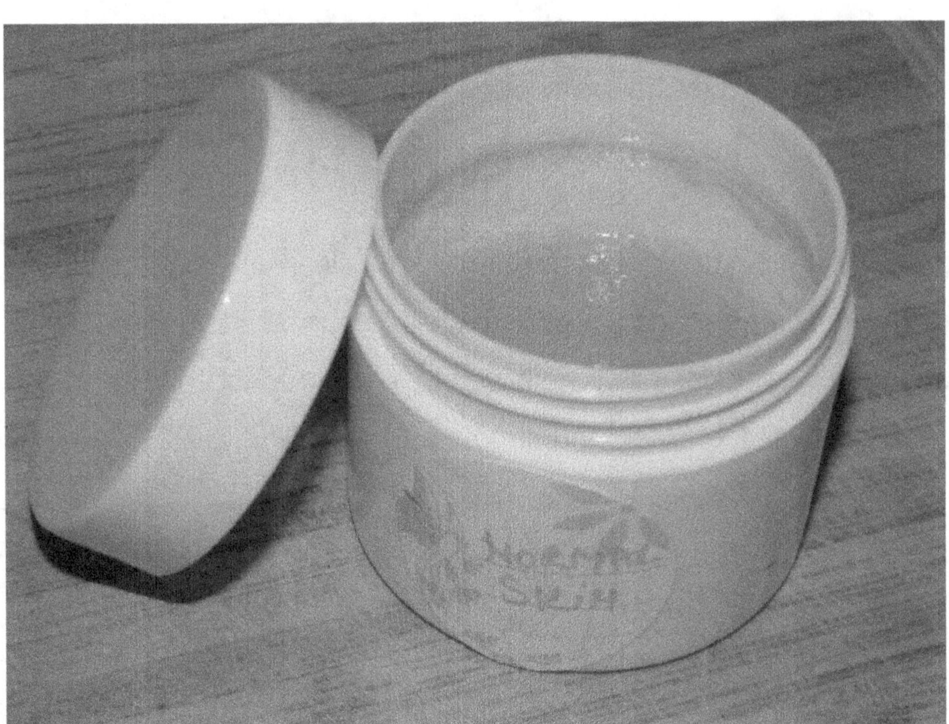

Facial Moisturizer for Oily Skin

When I first discovered the natural cosmetic products I was fighting with an oily skin and no matter what I did, my condition wouldn't improve. I have tried all the lotions I could find that promised me a nice face with no oily traces. But the result was the same: my face kept shining :) And not because it was very healthy and radiant...

When I started researching for natural remedies, I noticed that almost all the lotions were based on oils and butters. How could I put oil on my oily skin? I hesitated a lot before doing this step.

Until I found a perfectly logic explanation (logic for me :)) that convinced me I should give it a try: the oil used in the facial lotion has the power to dissolve the excess oil that is stuck on the pores.

If you use a natural facial moisturizer after you do the oil cleansing method, it is even better. The oil cleansing method is like detoxifying your face by massaging it with a combination of olive and castor oil, followed by placing a hot towel on your face. This way, your face will feel clean and happy.

You will need:

- 1,7 oz sweet almond oil
- 0,7 oz rosewater
- 2 tbsp jojoba wax/beeswax
- 5 drops Vitamin E oil
- 3-4 drops Grapefruit/Tea Tree essential oil

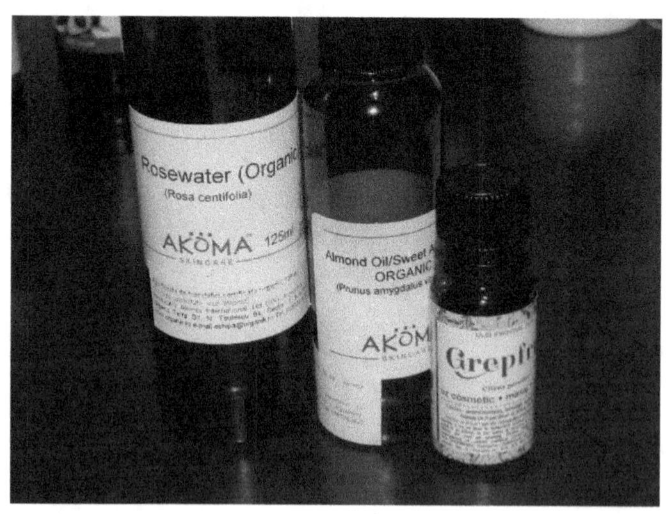

Directions:

1. Combine the sweet almond oil and the wax in a jar.
2. Place the jar into a pan half filled with water.

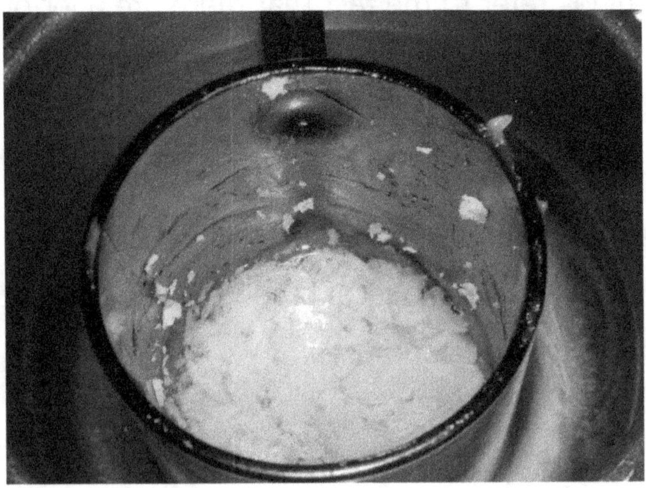

3. Use low heat to melt the wax.
4. After this is done remove the jar from the heat.
5. Let it cool for a while, stirring continuously.
6. Slowly pour the rosewater and keep stirring until the lotion becomes smooth.
7. Add the Vitamin E oil and the essential oil and mix well.
8. Use as your daily cream.
9. Store in a dry container.
10. Keep in the fridge or in a dark, cool place.

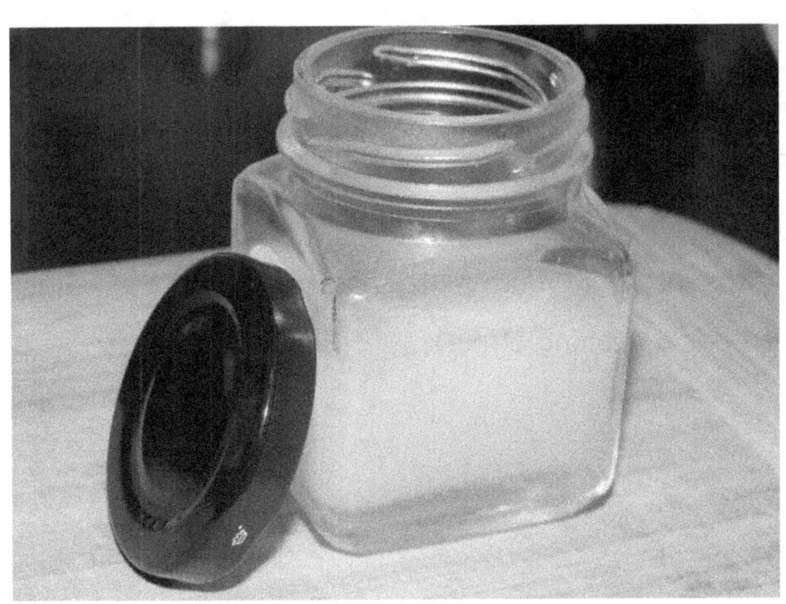

Olive Oil Night Cream

I've heard so many good things and bad things about the olive oil lately that I am very careful when I buy it. All the bad things refer to the fact that there are a lot of people and companies which forge olive oil by putting all kinds of additives into it to yield a lower price.

For this particular reason I pay very much attention when I buy this kind of oil. I've made my last acquisition from Greece, last year, from a local producer. I consider it's safer this way. We use it both for food and cosmetic purposes.

Olive oil's use for beauty dates back hundreds of years. The good thing about it is that it forms a barrier at the epidermis' level that keeps the moisture inside. This is way this night cream is so nourishing and hydrating.

Isn't it fabulous how you can take of your skin using only natural ingredients? I've been preparing my own cosmetic products for few years now and I'm still amazed by the fact that each day I discover new ingredients and also new ways of combining them.

For this recipe, you will need:

- 1 tbsp coconut oil
- ¼ cup extra virgin olive oil
- ¼ tsp Vitamin E oil (2 capsules)
- 1 tsp beeswax/jojoba wax
- 5 drops Lavender essential oil (you may try another flavor, like Roman Chamomile, it also has a relaxing effect)

Directions:

1. Combine the oils and the wax in a glass recipient.

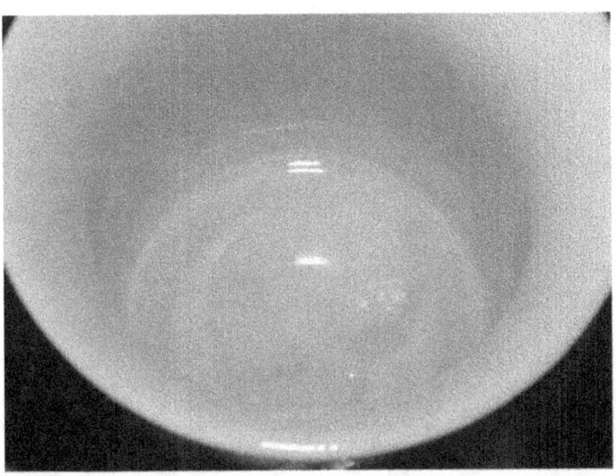

2. Place it in a pan half filled with water, over low heat.
3. Stir occasionally.
4. When the wax is melted, remove from heat.
5. Add the Vitamin E oil and the essential oil.

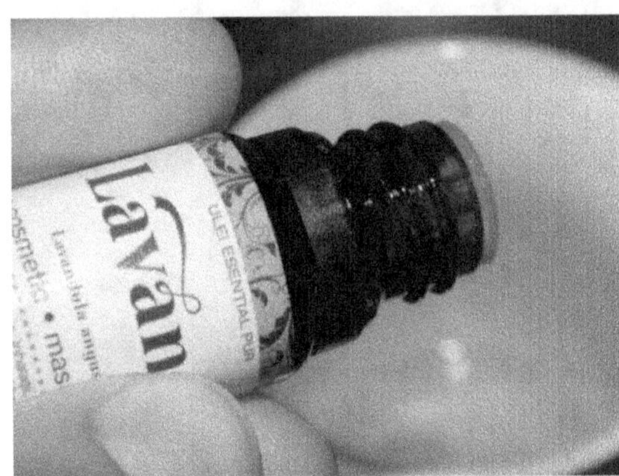

6. Pour the mixture in the storage container and let it cool until it solidifies.

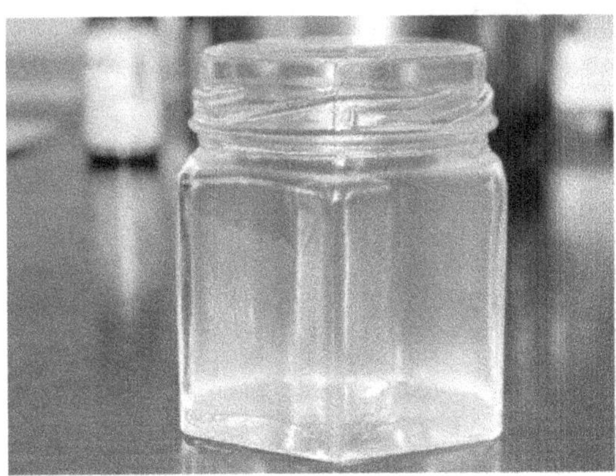

7. If you want a butter consistency, you may put it in the freezer until it starts to harden.

8. Take it out and mix it with a hand blender until it becomes fluffy.

9. Use it every night before going to bed.

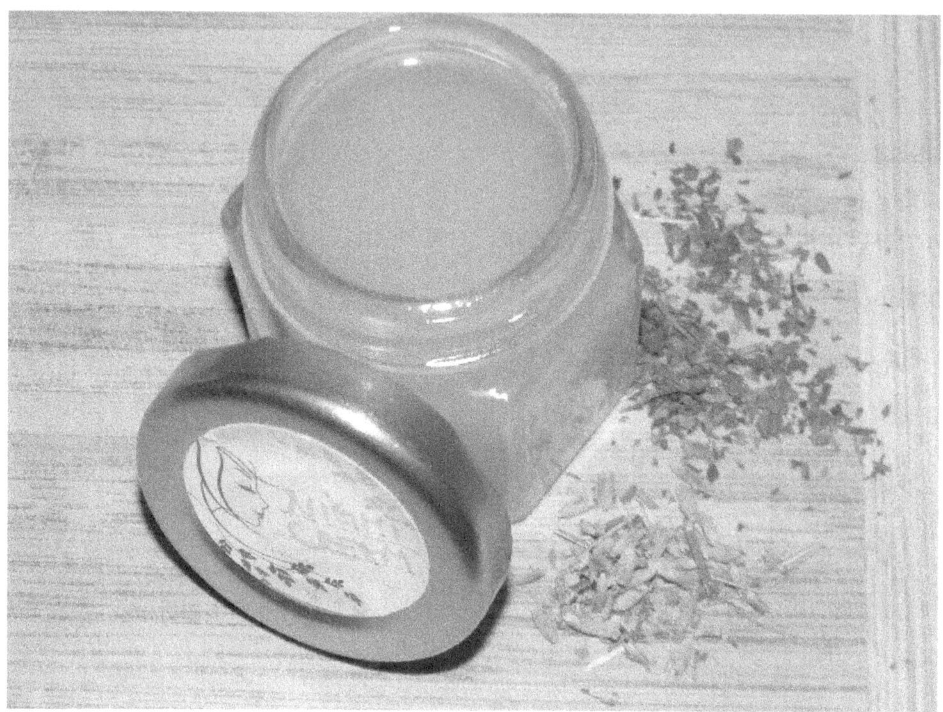

Strawberry Facial Moisturizer

A healthy glowing skin is probably one of the most desirable things of all women. If you already have it like this, it is good to preserve it. If not, you should try to get it.

A good intake of water can be the secret for this kind of brightness. Skin hydration is essential, and this can be achieved by using moisturizers but also through a proper daily intake of water to detoxify the body. Moisturizer acts as a protective layer for the skin, prevents wrinkles and accelerates cell renewal. Without moisturizing, skin can become wrinkled, dry and dull. The benefit of homemade moisturizer is that it will always be fresh, without parabens and other harmful substances.

And what can be better than to put food on your face? Like strawberries which, beside the fact that they are delicious and smell fabulous, bring the salicylic acid on your skin. And this acid has the power to remove the dead cells, reduce pores and brighten the skin.

You will need:
- 1 tbsp coconut oil
- 1 tbsp extra virgin olive oil
- 1 tbsp sunflower oil
- 2 tbsp strawberry puree
- 2 drops Vitamin E oil

Directions:

1. Combine all the oils.
2. If the coconut oil is solid you may place the oils jar in a bowl with warm water until the coconut melts.
3. Slowly add the puree and Vitamin E oil.
4. Mix until everything is well combined.

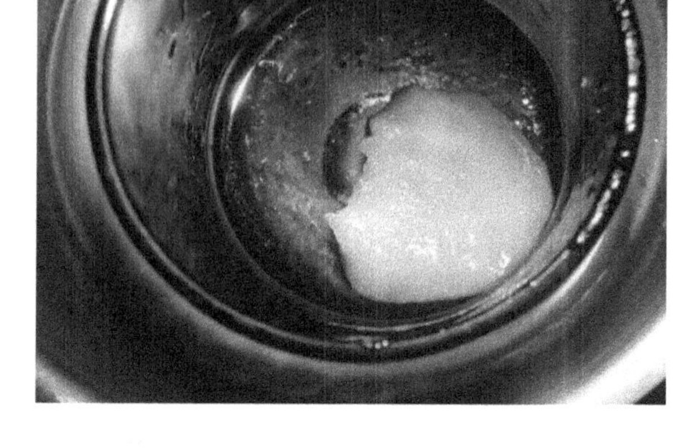

5. Vitamin E is a natural preservative, but the strawberry puree is quite perishable. This is why you should store your lotion in an airtight container.

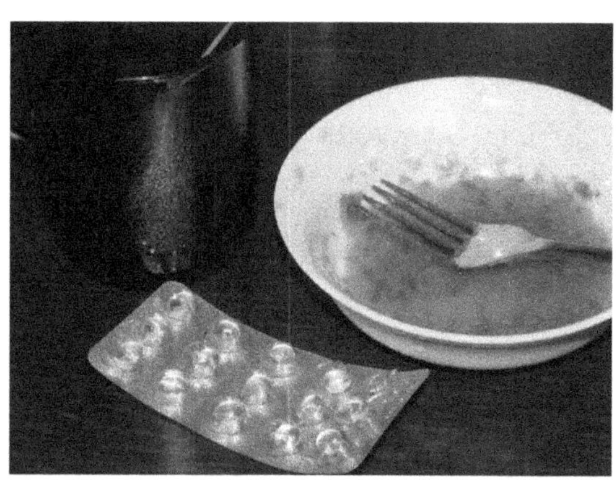

6. Keep it in the fridge until it's done.

The lotion is moisturizing, and it also can be used as face cleanser as it efficiently removes the make-up.

Enjoy your glowing skin and try more homemade lotions/creams!

Super Simple Facial Moisturizer

I know that there are many of you that don't want to start preparing homemade lotions fearing that it is too complicated and that it takes a lot of time. Well, I have good news for you: it is actually quite simple and there are a lot of recipes to choose from. Some of them are so easy to prepare that you start wondering why on earth have you ever bothered going to the store to buy some facial lotions when it is so comfortable to prepare them at home.

This recipe uses only three ingredients that can make wonders for your face: Coconut oil – extremely

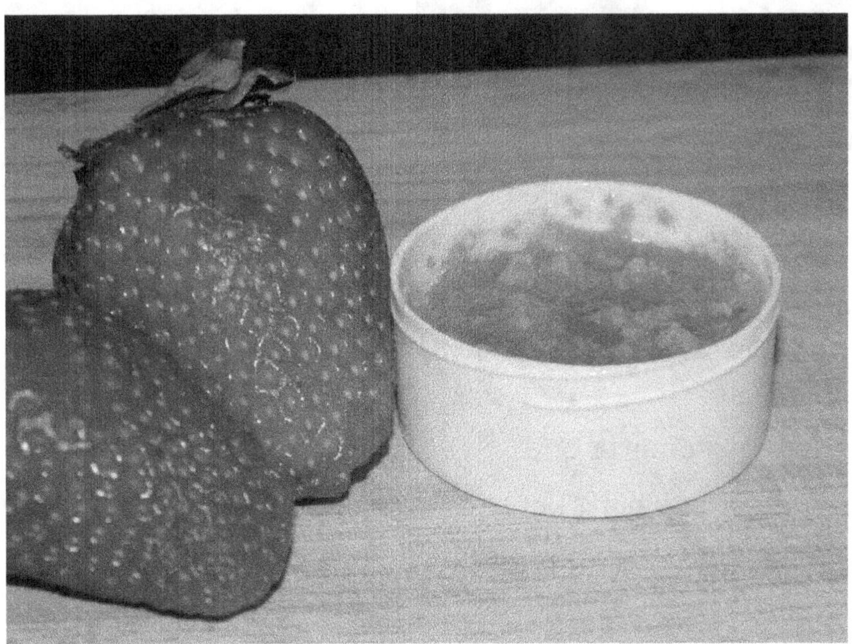

moisturizing with anti-aging properties. It also has anti-bacterial qualities and it can protect your skin from aggressive external agents.

Lavender essential oil – it has calming and relaxing properties and antioxidant effects

Vitamin E oil – has a healing effect, especially over scar tissues. It is also effective in skin blemishes and acne.

You will need:

- ½ cup coconut oil
- 12 drops Lavender essential oil
- 1 tsp Vitamin E oil

Directions:

1. Put the coconut oil in a jar.
2. Place the jar in a pan/bowl half filled with warm water.
3. Let the coconut oil melt.
4. Add the Vitamin E oil and the essential oil.
5. Now, you may pour the mixture in the storage container and let it cool.

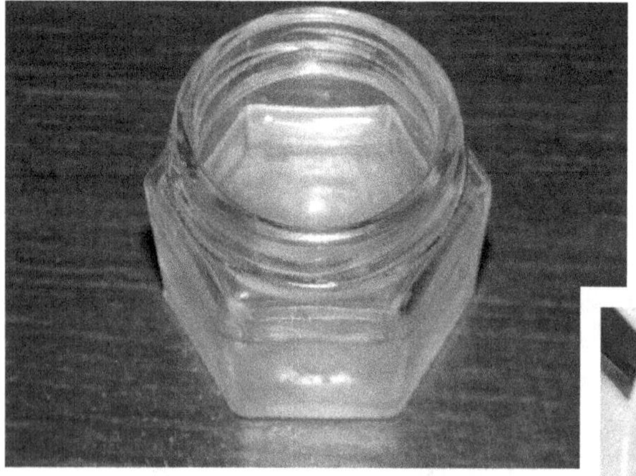

6. Or you may use a hand mixer or a small food processor to whip it until you get a butter consistency. It is all

up to you.

7. Keep the lotion in a dry, cool place.

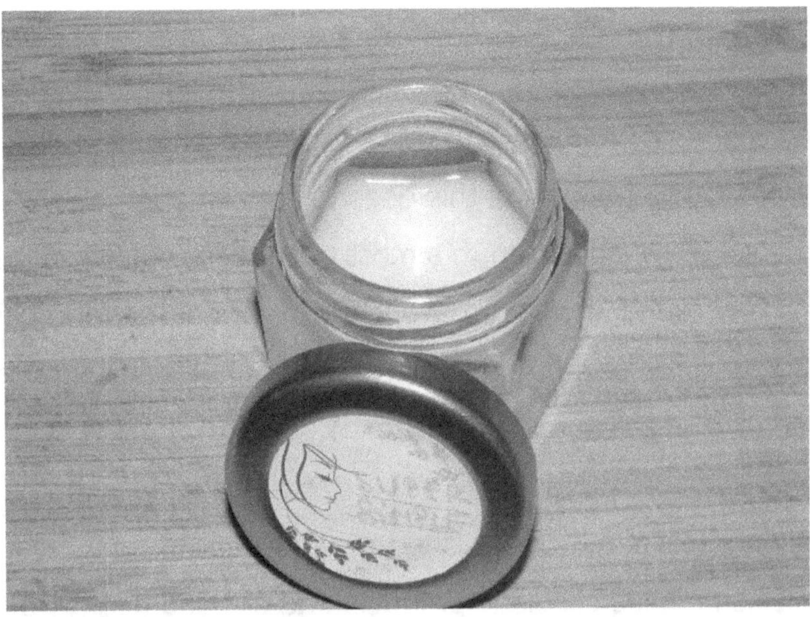

What can be easier than this? It is quite simple to prepare a facial moisturizer using only 3 ingredients, don't you think? Not to mention that it does wonders for your face. You should definitely try this at home!

Vanilla Face Cream

I love the smell of vanilla as it always reminds me of ice cream :) Oh yeah, I also love vanilla ice cream. But after all, who doesn't?

I enjoy flavoring my cosmetic products with this exquisite aroma, it feels like pampering myself when I use them. And this doesn't happen a lot lately. My life is like the bus from the song my kids listen to almost every day (you know "the wheels on the bus go round and round"): children, work, children, house work, children, going out in the park, children, etc... And sometimes in between I get to take a shower and use a scrub and a natural moisturizer :)

But I'm not complaining, this is the life I wished for and I get to do things that I enjoy, like preparing homemade cosmetic products and cooking healthy delicious foods.

And I would like to invite you to try at least one recipe for a homemade lotion/face cream, like the one below that smells like vanilla ice cream as I told you before. It contains only natural ingredients and it will do wonders for your skin.

You will need:

- 3 tbsp sweet almond oil
- 1/8 cup cocoa butter
- 1,5 tbsp shea butter
- 1 tbsp coconut oil
- 1/3 cup rosewater
- ¼ tsp Vitamin E oil
- 0,5 tbsp beeswax/jojoba wax
- 1/6 cup aloe vera gel
- 0,5 tsp vanilla extract

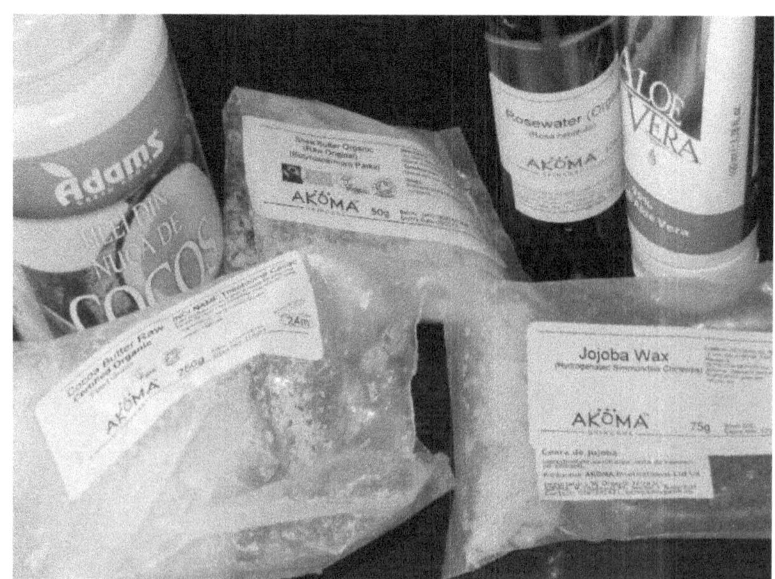

Directions:

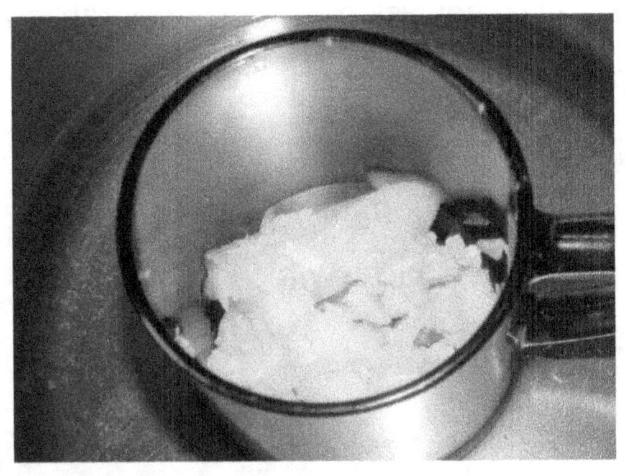

1. Combine the cocoa and shea butter and the coconut oil with the wax in glass jar.
2. Place the jar in a pan half filled with water.
3. Turn the heat on low and let the pan there until the wax melts.
4. Remove it from heat and set aside to cool a little bit.
5. Pour the floral water in the aloe gel and mix well.
6. Transfer the oil mixture to a food processor and add the sweet almond oil.
7. Slowly mix in the aloe vera gel, then add all the other ingredients.
8. Blend until fluffy.
9. Enjoy the facial moisturizer!

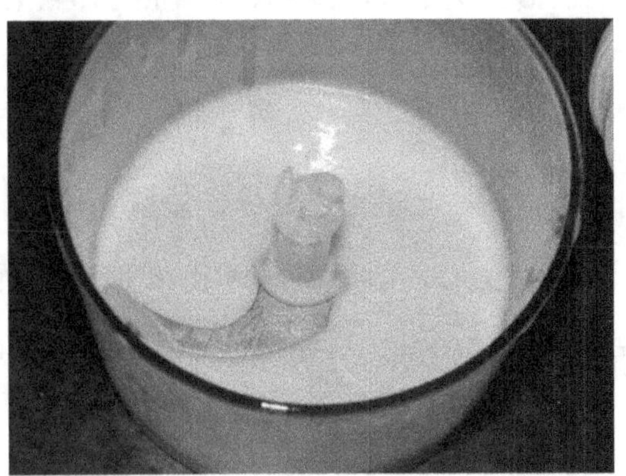

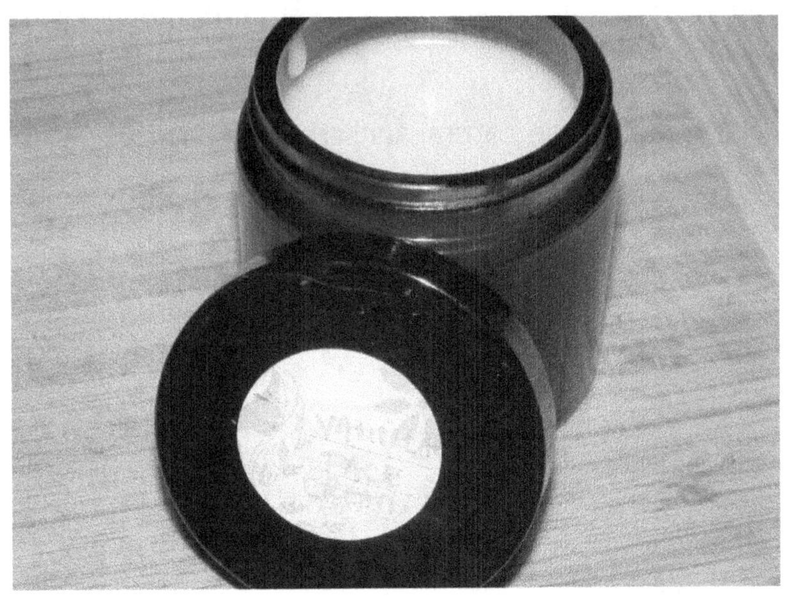

Natural Sunscreens

Spending too long in the sun is extremely harmful to your skin. It can accelerate the visible signs of aging and significantly increase your risk of contracting skin cancer.

While store bought solutions may seem like a viable solution for protecting yourself from the sun, they actually contain many dangerous chemicals which rapidly absorb into your body through your skin.

So, what's the solution?

Fortunately, it's quite a simple one…use natural ingredients to make your own highly effective sunscreens.

This section will show you how to make some simple all-natural sunscreens along with some completely natural bronzers. All of the tutorials use protective and healing natural ingredients such as beeswax, coconut oil, coffee and mango butter.

For each tutorial, you get:
-   A list of the ingredients you'll need to prepare the natural sunscreen or bronzer
-   Step by step text instructions describing how to prepare the natural sunscreen or bronzer
-   Photos showing you how to prepare the natural sunscreen or bronzer

So, let's get started making some natural sun protection!

Castor Oil Repellant

When the sun is shining, my kids always ask me: "When are we going to the seaside?" In fact, tomorrow we will be leaving. And my boy keeps asking me: "Is today tomorrow? When will tomorrow come? " :)

Since they are in such a hurry, I thought to myself that I should be prepared and I started packing 2 days ago. Not because I have too many bags, but because they keep searching through the suitcases when they see something of interest: like a toy or a water pistol or a ball.

And, if you have kids, you know that they don't take out only the object they want, but ten others also. I have to put them together again and again. It's like a never ending game. Which they enjoy. I don't.

So, I thought I have to be prepared for the sun rays, too. I really don't enjoy using common sunscreen as it contains a lot of chemicals which are absorbed very quickly. I prepare my own and I will show you my favorite recipe below.

You Will Need:

- ✓ 1/2 cup calendula infused oil
- ✓ 1/4 cup coconut oil
- ✓ 1/4 cup beeswax pastilles
- ✓ 2 tbsp shea butter
- ✓ 2 tbsp zinc oxide
- ✓ 1 tsp raspberry seed oil
- ✓ Essential oils of choice (I use lavender and mint)

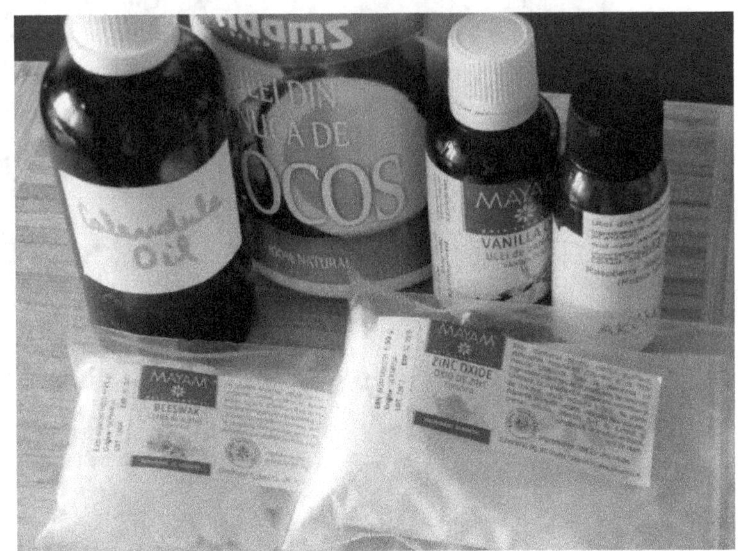

Directions:

1. Melt together the calendula infused oil, shea butter, coconut oil and the beeswax pastilles in a jar.

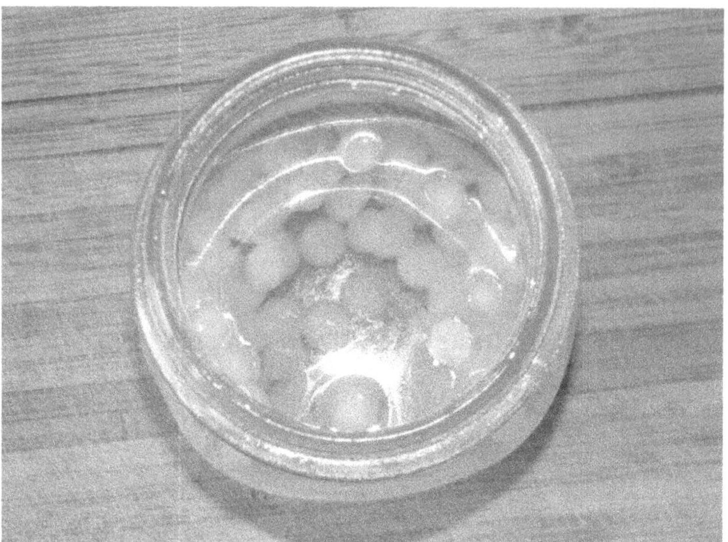

2. Use a double boiler or place the jar in a pan with hot water.

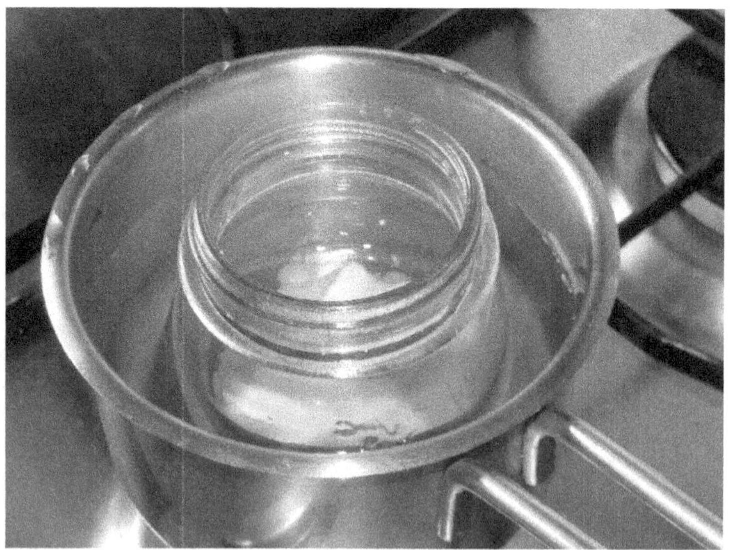

3. Remove from heat.
4. Add the raspberry seed oil.
5. Mix in the zinc oxide. Be careful to wear a mask so you don't inhale the powder. Stir well for the zinc oxide to be evenly distributed.

6. Add the essential oils and stir again.

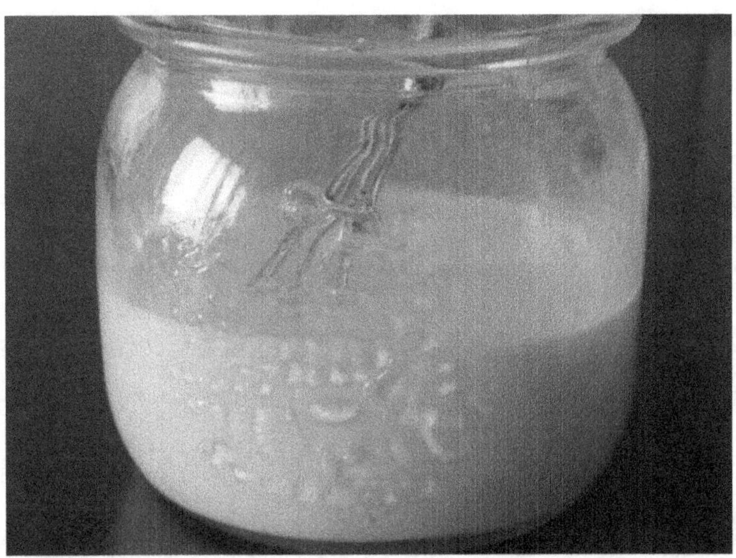

7. Pour the mixture into a clean container and let it cool and harden.

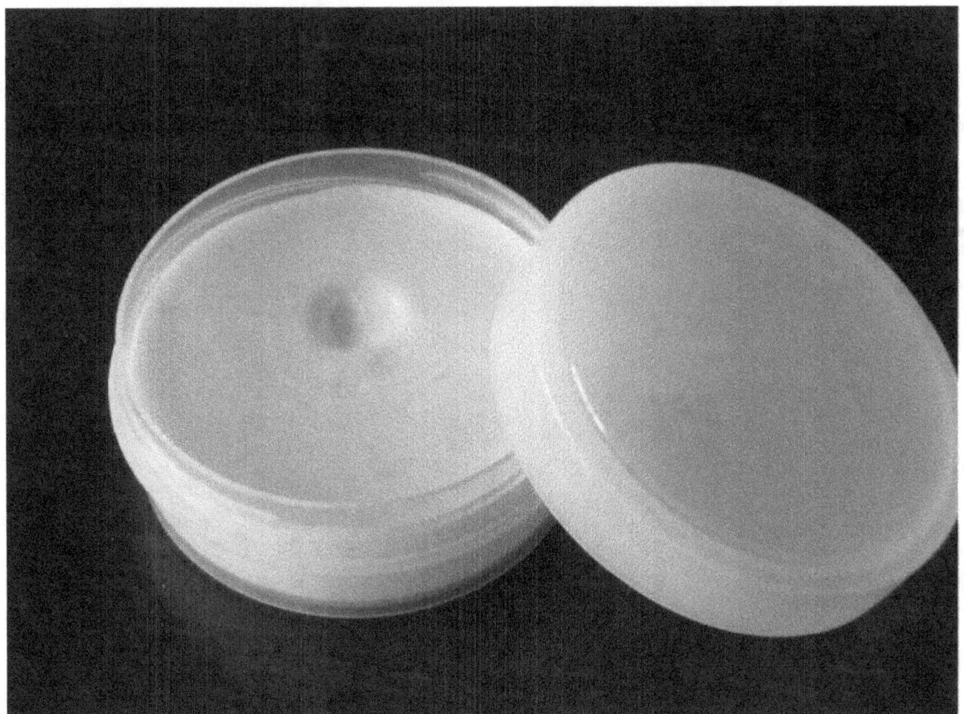

Cocoa Bronzer

One good reason for using a bronzer is when the sun is shining, and you haven't got any hope to go to the seaside as soon as you would wish. Or that you don't have enough time to go to the pool. Or that your skin is very sensitive, and you don't want to expose it to direct sun rays. Either way, using a bronzer is one of the healthiest choices you have. If the bronzer is natural, of course.

If you apply it all over your body take care that it might leave stains on your clothes or bedding before it is completely dry. Drying time varies, but it may last from 15 to 30 minutes.

Exfoliate before applying the bronzer. It adheres to dead skin cells and there are areas where the stratum corneum is thicker (knees, elbows, feet, neck). You can exfoliate your skin with a loofah when taking a shower or you may use a homemade scrub.

Do you need shaving? Do it before applying the bronzer. Waxing (or other forms of hair removal, like shaving) may affect the quality of the bronze and shorten the duration it will look natural on the skin.

You Will Need:

- ✓ Premade white lotion
- ✓ Cocoa powder

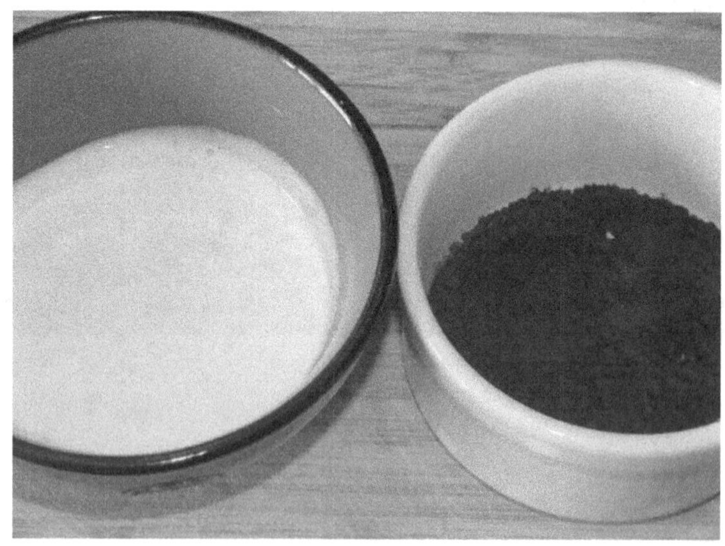

Directions:

1. Adjust the quantities taking into consideration the area you want to apply the bronzer on.
2. You may start with 1/2 cup lotion.
3. Mix in 1/3 cup cocoa powder. Use a strain for the cocoa so you don't get any clumps. Mix well and test it on your skin.
4. Adjust the color depending on the desired bronze intensity. Add cocoa little by little until you reach the perfect shade.
5. If you want a deep tan, you should use it every day.
6. Apply over your entire body. Make sure you do it evenly because you don't want different colors on your legs and hands.

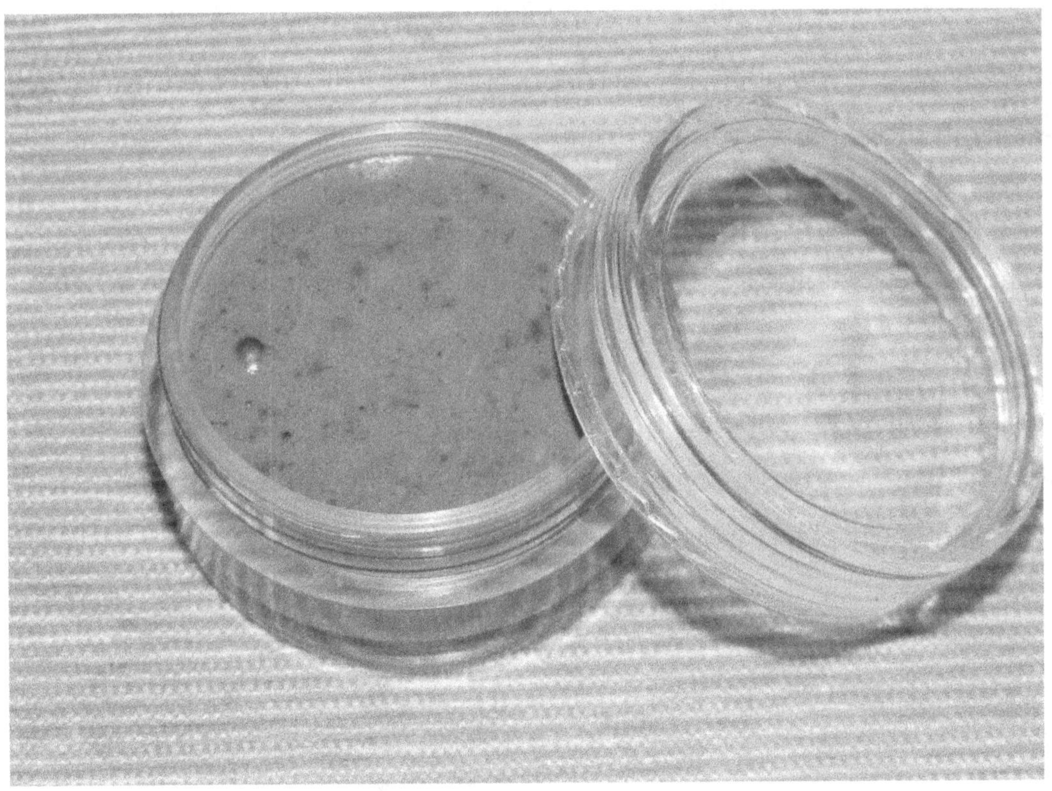

Coconut Oil Bronzer

It is proven: a tan obtained with a bronzer is the only way you can have a coppery color without putting your skin (or health) in danger due to unprotected sun exposure. But as anyone who used a bronzer may tell you, getting a uniform tan is not so simple.

It may even be difficult to obtain, especially for the beginners. The good news is that there are some tips that you can use for obtaining a radiant tan.

The color obtained with the bronzer depends on individual body chemistry. If a bronzer looks natural on one of your friends, this does not mean it will have the same effect on your skin. You must be patient. If you're going to get all your body browny, the procedure can last more than 30 minutes.

After your take a shower and the skin completely dry, apply a thin layer of moisturizer in areas where you apply the bronzer. This step will make it easier to be applied, especially in those places with dry skin.

If you want to apply the tanner only on your face and neck, do it preferably as the last step in routine care, taking care to evenly distribute in difficult areas (nose, ears, neck).

Natural bronzers don't leave orange stains, but you may get dirty clothes. For the next recipe you will use coconut oil so make sure you wait enough for it to be absorbed by the skin so it doesn't leave greasy marks.

You Will Need:

- ✓ Coconut oil
- ✓ Cocoa powder

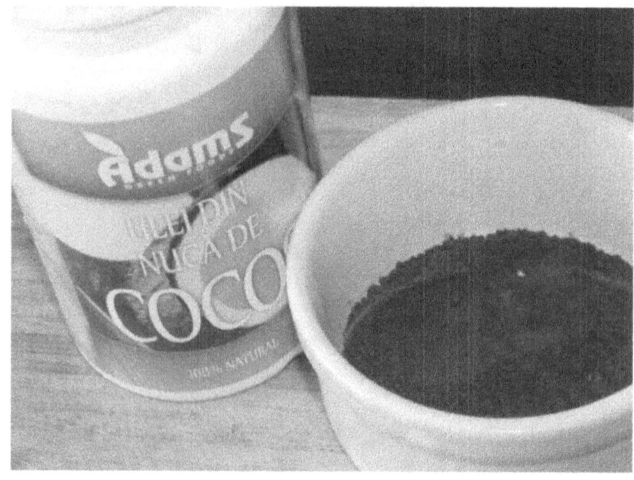

Directions:

1. If you need a bronzer for the entire body, use a larger quantity of coconut oil (approximately 1/2 cup).
2. Mix in the cocoa powder and whisk well. You don't need any clumps in your bronzer.
3. Add the cocoa gradually until you reach the desired color.
4. Apply daily for a nice tan.

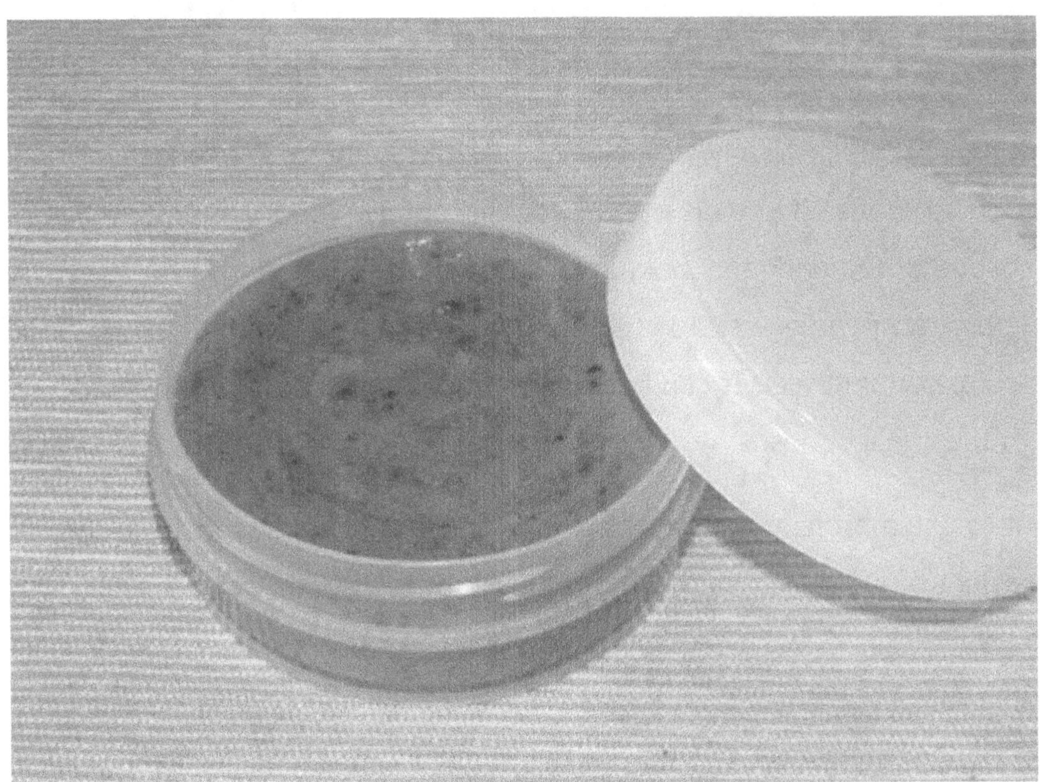

Coffee Tanner

A bronzer is a little beauty trick that you can call to have a skin kissed by the sun and you do not necessarily need to go to the beach. To achieve the desired effect, however, you must know how to choose the tanner according to your skin tone and how to apply it correctly.

You will want a bronzer if you have either too white skin or you simply want to get that sexy copper color that is worn especially in summer.

A bronzer can be your friend or foe ... depends if you know how to use it.

And although it can be an ally in any woman's beauty bag, a bronzer is a rather problematic product because if you do not choose it properly, you risk either making your skin too orange or too dark and look unnatural. And the way of applying it counts too. The bronzer can be used to create a nicer tanned look or just to highlight and sculpt certain traits. It can be used on face, neck and body and can replace blush to the cheekbones.

When you want to use a bronzer you must pay attention to several aspects so that you choose the right one. You should have a tanner that is a shade or two darker than your skin. White skin looks good with a peach, pink or honey-colored bronzer, olive skin is beautifully highlighted with a copper-colored bronzer and darker skin accepts darker tanners. If you still have problems in making the best bronzer, guide yourself by the color of your foundation or face powder.

The best choice ever is a homemade bronzer. This is the only way you will get the perfect shade and you will be able to do this by adjusting the color little by little.

You Will Need:

- ✓ Ground coffee
- ✓ Premade white lotion

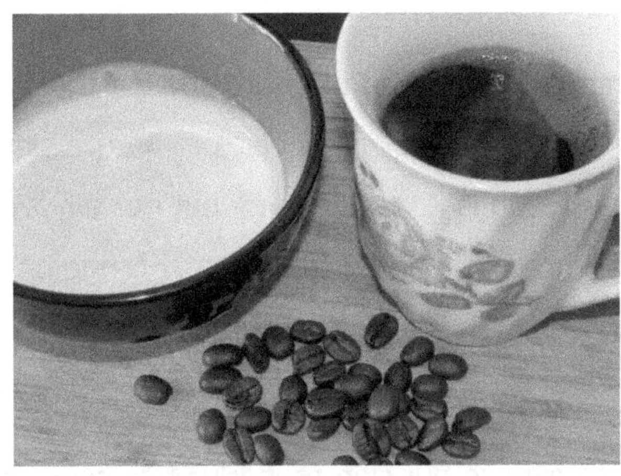

Directions:

1. If you need a bronzer for the entire body, use a larger quantity of coconut oil (approximately 1/2 cup).
2. Combine the lotion with the coffee and mix well. Add coffee until you get your desired color.
3. Store the mixture in a spray bottle and apply daily.

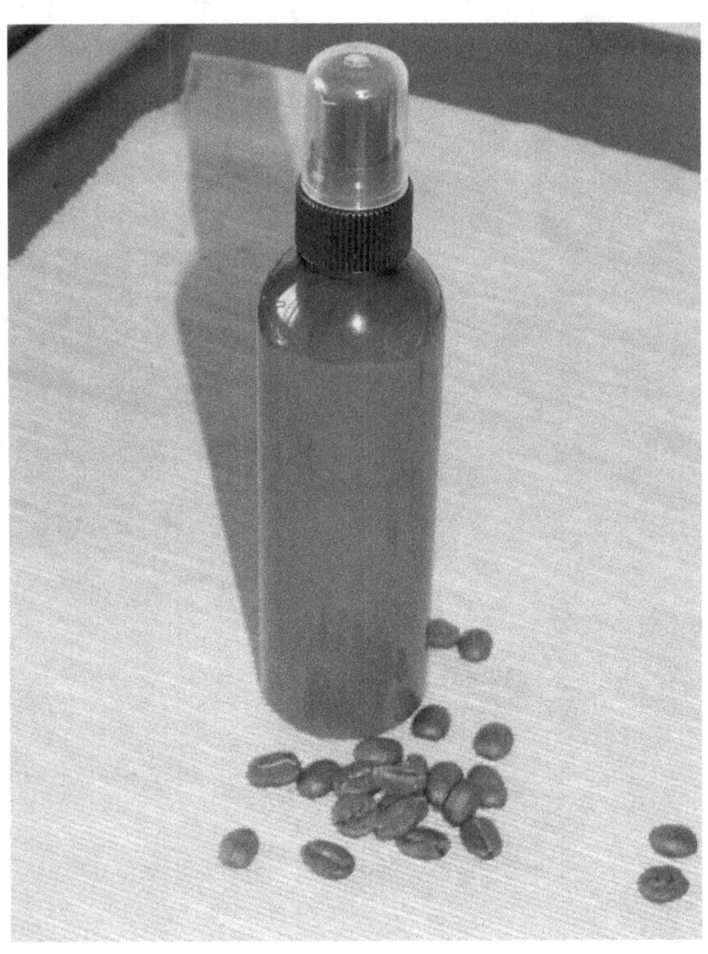

Homemade Sunscreen

We are increasingly urged to guard against the sun for various reasons: we get burn, we may develop skin cancer, premature skin aging, etc. But what no one tells us is that the sun is not the enemy but our ally. Sun helps us produce vitamin D whose absence in the body can cause a range of diseases, but also an increased risk of cancer.

This does not mean you have to sit all day on the beach. It's just that we should not be afraid to expose our skin properly or to cover ourselves with sun protection creams from sunrise until sunset. It is best to protect ourselves with appropriate clothes and hats and use sunscreen during the time we stay at the beach or perform prolonged outdoor activities and we are not protected by clothing.

You should use only natural sunscreen, which offers mineral protection. This acts like a barrier for the sun rays and it is not absorbed by the skin. In fact mineral sun blockers, like zinc oxide, are like a mirror which reflects the UVA and UVB rays.

You Will Need:

- ✓ 1/4 cup shea butter
- ✓ 1/4 cup coconut oil
- ✓ 1/4 cup sesame oil
- ✓ 2 tbsp beeswax pastilles
- ✓ 1 tsp red raspberry seed oil
- ✓ 1-2 tbsp zinc oxide
- ✓ 1 tsp carrot seed oil
- ✓ 20 drops Lavender essential oil

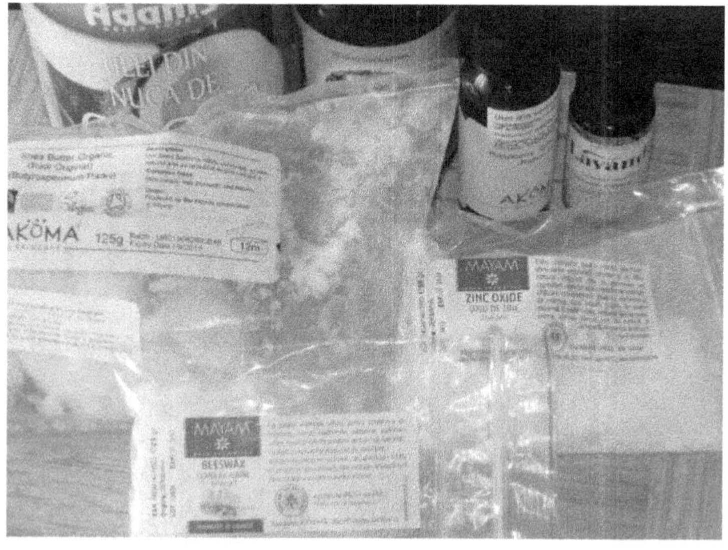

Directions:

1. Take a glass jar and combine the following ingredients: shea butter, coconut oil, sesame oil, beeswax pastilles.

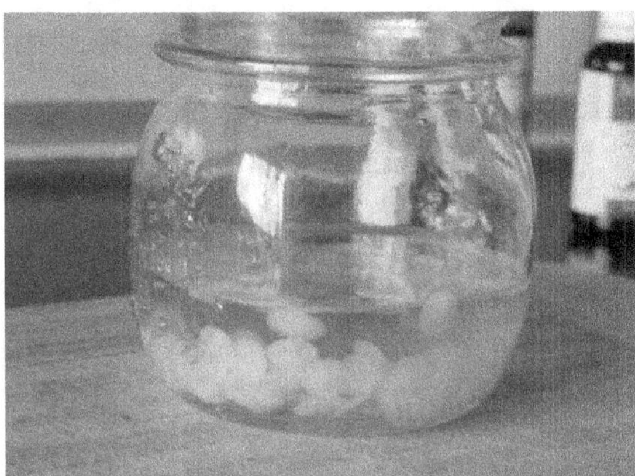

2. Melt them on a pan with hot water, over low heat. Make sure you don't boil the butter and oils as they lose their beneficial properties.

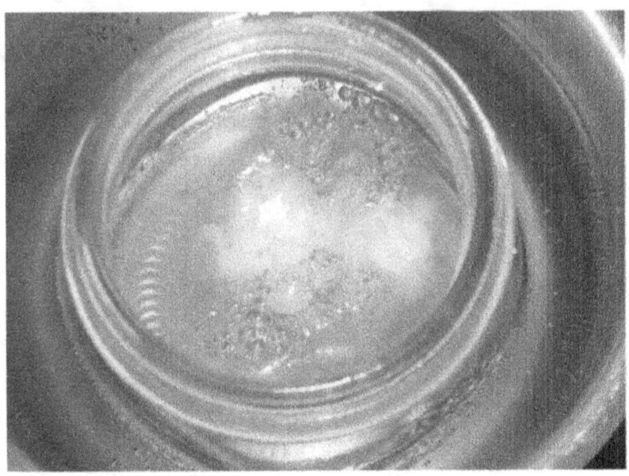

3. Once they have melted, remove from heat.

4. Add the red raspberry seed oil and the carrot seed oil. Stir well.

5. Mix in the zinc oxide, being carefully not to inhale the powder. You may wear a mask to avoid this.

6. Stir well again so the zinc oxide is evenly distributed.

7. Add the essential oil and mix again.

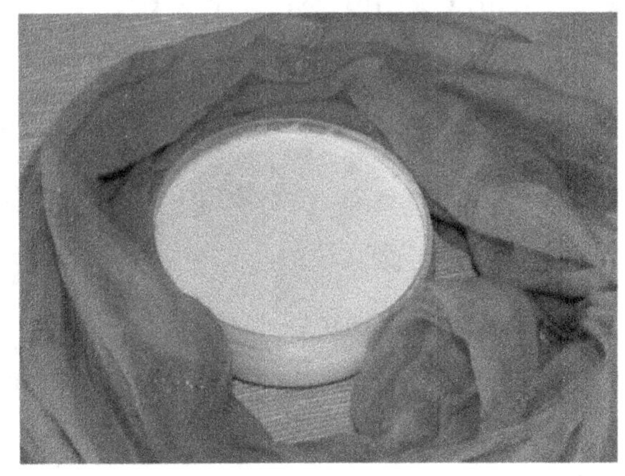

8. Transfer to a clean container and apply when needed.

Low SPF Sunscreen

Sun is life. Yes, I know it sounds a little poetic, but it is the truth. Without sun and light, many of the things that surround us wouldn't exist. Have you ever noticed that in a dense and dark forest the grass does not grow at all, while in bright clearings or in places where the sun creeps a lot of flowers and plants grow? This is true for humans also. Isn't it right that you have a better mood in a sunny day?

But as we all know, sun protection is a very controversial topic. I've read lots of reviews: it's better to expose ourselves to the sun, but with sun protection; it's not good to expose ourselves to the sun after 10:00 AM; sunlight can cause skin cancer; and so on.

There are many questions and many studies in this area.

Many researchers have found that natural means of protection from the sun, such as coconut oil, sesame oil, shea butter are actually more effective than store bought alternatives. Plus, they do not contain toxic ingredients like these common lotions do.

So, why don't we do the same? You may choose among hundreds of recipes. Here is one for a low SPF sunscreen suitable for the days when the sun is not burning.

You Will Need:

- ✓ 1/2 cup coconut oil (SPF 4-6)
- ✓ 1 tbsp red raspberry seed oil (SPF 10-15)
- ✓ 1 tbsp vanilla oil (for its delicate scent)
- ✓ 1/4 cup shea butter (SPF 4-6)

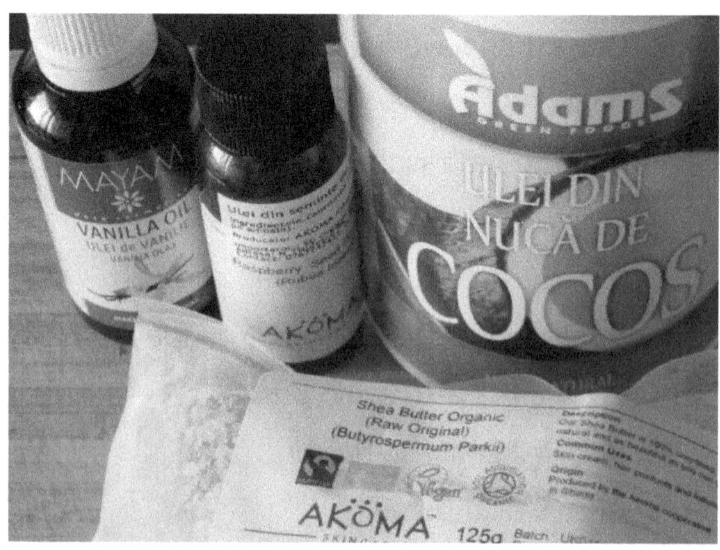

Directions:

1. Melt the shea butter together with the coconut oil using a double boiler or a pan with hot water.
2. Remove from heat and add the raspberry and vanilla oil. Stir well.
3. You will get a lotion with about 20-25 SPF.
4. It is also a great moisturizer so apply every time you want to.

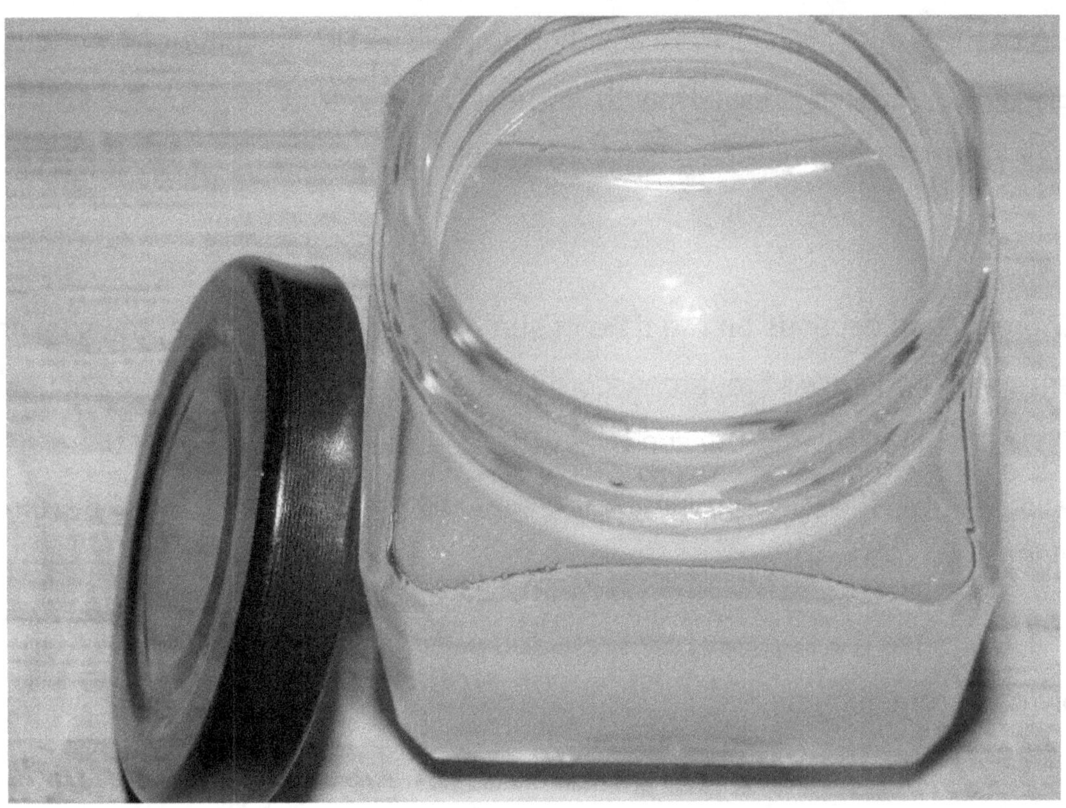

Mango Butter Sunscreen

When talking about sun exposure, we should take a look at the vitamin D production. The human body cannot produce this vitamin other than through sun exposure. "Ultraviolet radiation (UVB) are really essential for a robust health. The idea that we must protect ourselves from the sun all the time is wrong and unhealthy.

Sun phobia explains why so many people are suffering from conditions related to deprivation of the sun. "(Michael F. Holick, PhD, MD - The UV Advantage, The Medical Breakthrough That Shows How to Harness the Power of The Sun for Your Health , J.Boylston & Co., Publishers, New York, 2003 x).

Vitamin D production depends on the time of sun exposure, how vertical the sunlight is, the hemisphere where we are, etc. According to researchers, to produce enough vitamin D we should expose to the sun rays without protective creams 2-3 times a week just between 10:00AM – 3:00PM, just enough so our skin doesn't become red (10-20 minutes maximum).

Outside these periods the skin must be protected with natural sunscreen which are based only on natural ingredients. Beside this exposure, avoid direct sunlight between 10:00-16:00.

The sun is the same as a few years ago, although there are opinions how it would be more dangerous. On the contrary, some researchers argue that some holes in the ozone layer have been plugged.

Otherwise the residents of equatorial countries should all have cancer. But studies show that this disease may be caused by the chemical ingredients from the conventional sunscreen.

Here is a recipe for a natural sunscreen you may prepare at home.

You Will Need:

- ✓ 1 oz oil blend (sweet almond and calendula oil)
- ✓ 1 oz mango butter
- ✓ 1 oz beeswax
- ✓ 30 drops essential oils of choice (avoid citrus ones, they are photo toxic)
- ✓ 0.36 oz zinc oxide powder

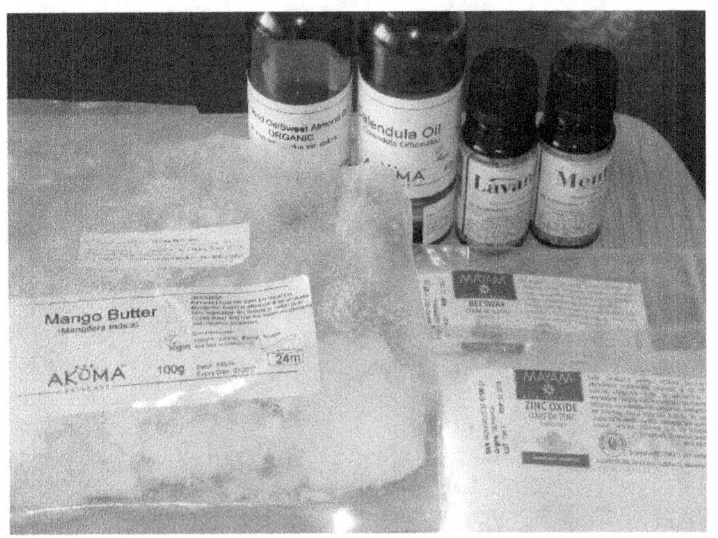

Directions:

1. Combine the oils, mango butter and the beeswax in a glass jar.

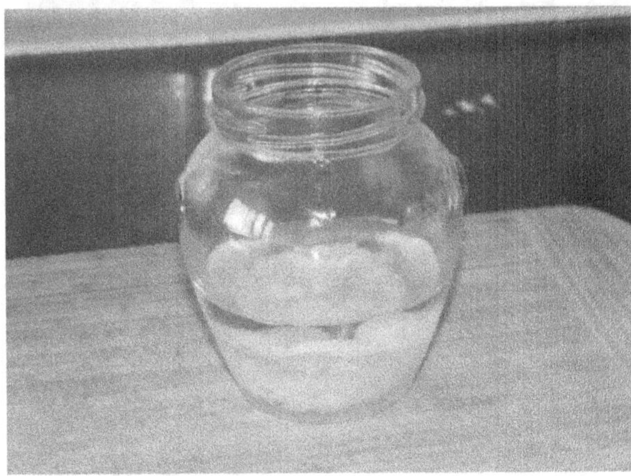

2. Melt them over low heat. Use a pan with hot water.

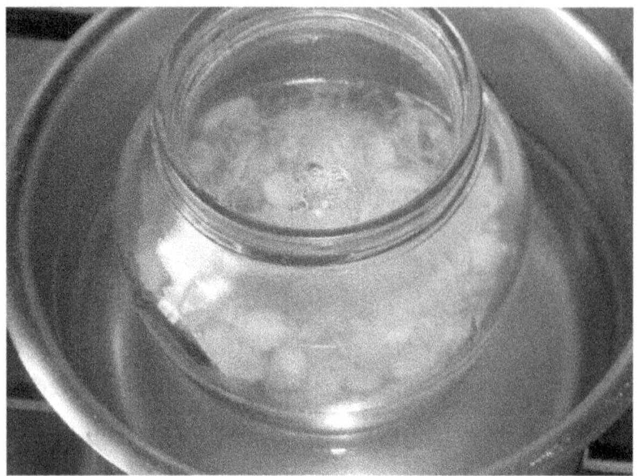

3. Add the essential oils, then mix in the zinc oxide. You may want to wear a mask so you don't inhale the powder. Make sure it is evenly distributed.
4. Store in a clean container and reapply often when you are at the beach or pool.

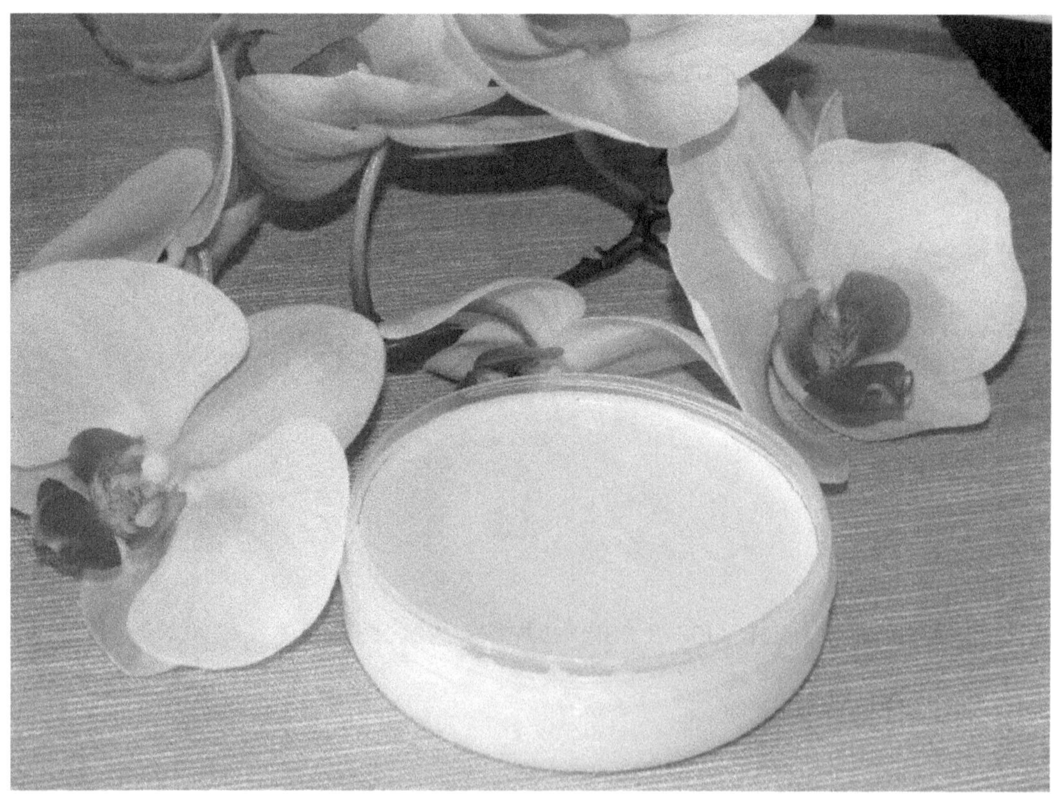

Natural Sunscreen

A prolonged exposure to sunlight can lead to wrinkles. Repeated sunburns increase the risk of skin cancer.

The sun produces many kinds of rays, but we are concerned in particular with ultraviolet A (UVA) and ultraviolet B (UVB). UVB rays are the ones that stimulate the production of vitamin D which is actually good for us. UVA are seen as the main risk factor in causing skin cancer. Experts say it is best to expose ourselves to the sun until the skin gets a slight shade of pink. Vitamin D production also occurs in this interval.

Of course, it depends on skin color too. After this period, the body no longer produces vitamin D, the maximum of one day being reached. After the skin gets this color it is advisable to stop direct exposure to the sun because of the risk of severe burns. Most common sunscreens protect only against UVB rays, which is nonsense considering that they are responsible for producing vitamin D.

UVB rays reach their maximum strength at noon and filter quite easily if it is cloudy. Unfortunately, the same thing doesn't happen with the UVA which are burning even if the weather is cloudy. UVB don't have power in the evening unlike the UVA.

The best thing you can do is to use a natural sunscreen which acts like a mirror and reflects the sun rays and to limit the exposure during the hours when the sun has maximum power.

Here is a homemade sunscreen recipe.

You Will Need:

- ✓ 1 oz emulsifying olive wax
- ✓ 8 oz sweet almond oil
- ✓ 2-7 tbsp zinc oxide powder
- ✓ 30 drops lavender essential oil

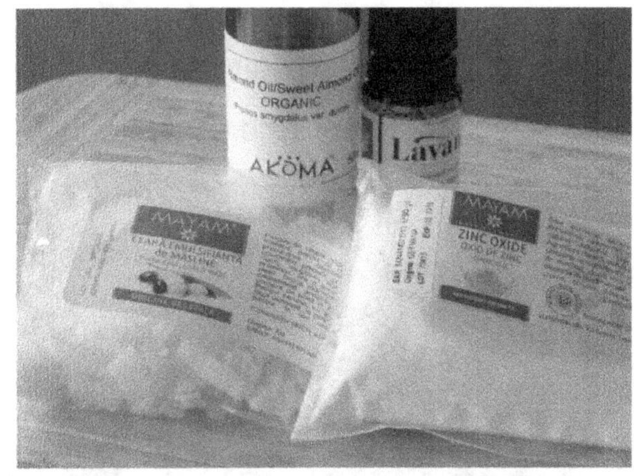

Directions:

1. Add the wax to a glass jar.

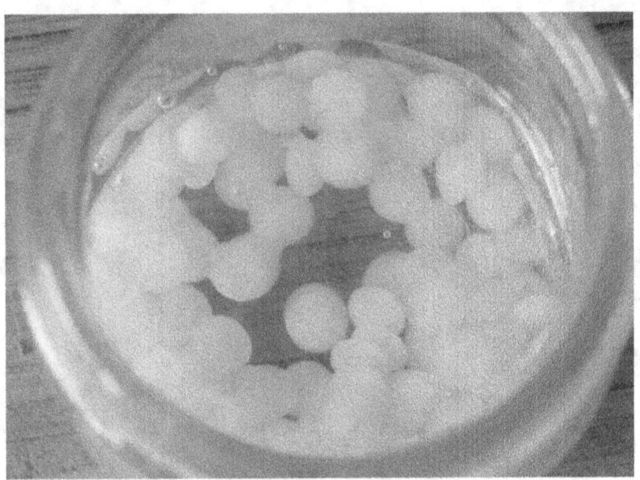

2. Melt the wax over low heat.

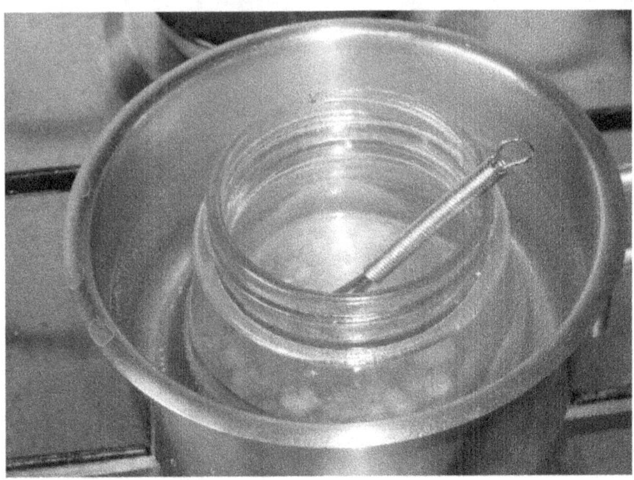

3. Add the sweet almond oil and stir well.

4. Pour the lavender oil and mix again.

5. Add the zinc oxide (the more you use, the higher the SPF – starting from 20-25) and make sure it is evenly distributed.

6. Reapply often, especially after taking a bath.

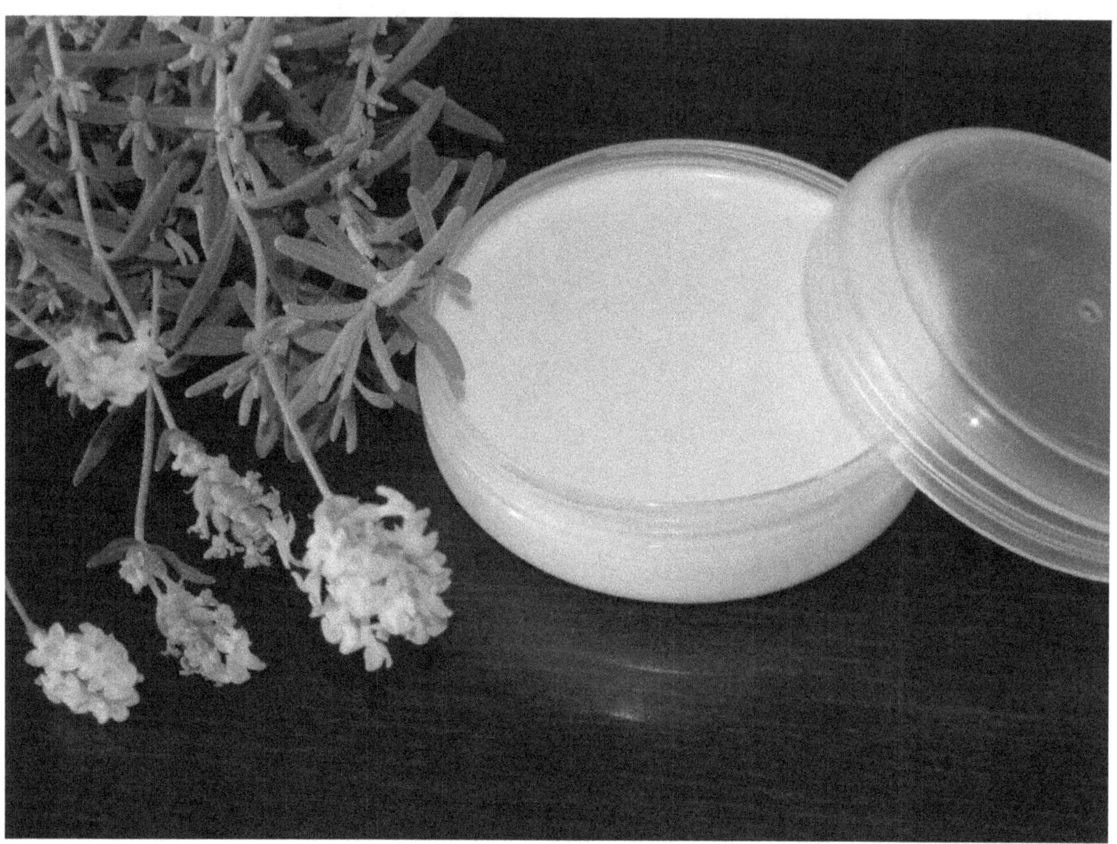

The skin is our largest organ, so everything we put on it is absorbed in 60%. Most of the ingredients contained in conventional sunscreens are chemicals which can disrupt endocrine function, increase the risk of cancer and lead to many other diseases. In fact, reports show that since the appearance of trade sun lotions, the skin cancer rate has increased.

In a document from 2007, FDA showed that by using sunscreen products we cannot prevent skin cancer. This even may increase the risk for its occurrence. This happens for a variety of reasons, including that they block UVB rays, leading to a deficiency of vitamin D. It is also stated that vitamin A and its derivatives used in conventional products become toxic when they are exposed to sunlight.

Natural sunscreen is based on mineral filters which do not absorb rays, but they reflect them. In addition, they do not contain harmful chemical ingredients.

Another thing we should consider for a healthy skin and tan is food. No one can deny that diet plays an essential role for the health of our skin. The old adage "you are what you eat" is very true. Food is the fuel on which the body works, so we must provide it with the right one. It is recommended eating foods rich in Omega-6: coconut oil, ghee, clarified butter, avocado and avocado oil, olive oil, etc in order to have a radiant skin.

If you want to try a natural sunscreen and you have some body lotions already prepared, here is one good recipe.

You Will Need:

- ✓ 3/4 cup homemade moisturizing lotion
- ✓ 3-4 tbsp zinc oxide (non-nano)

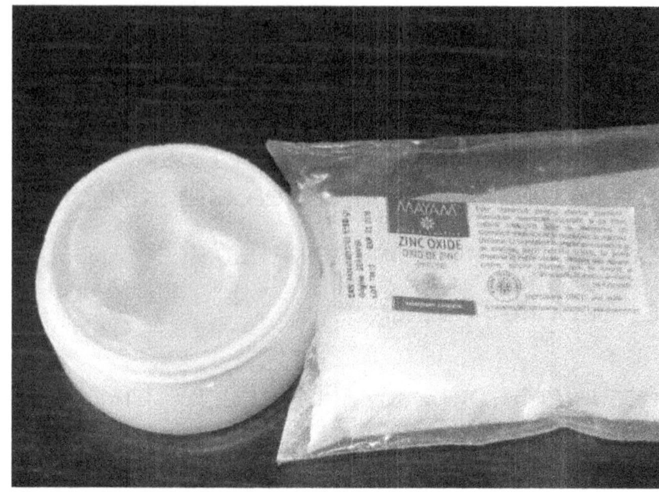

Directions:

1. Use a mask and mix the zinc oxide into the body lotion. You need the mask so you don't inhale the powder.
2. Stir to get the zinc oxide well distributed.
3. Take the lotion to the beach and apply often.

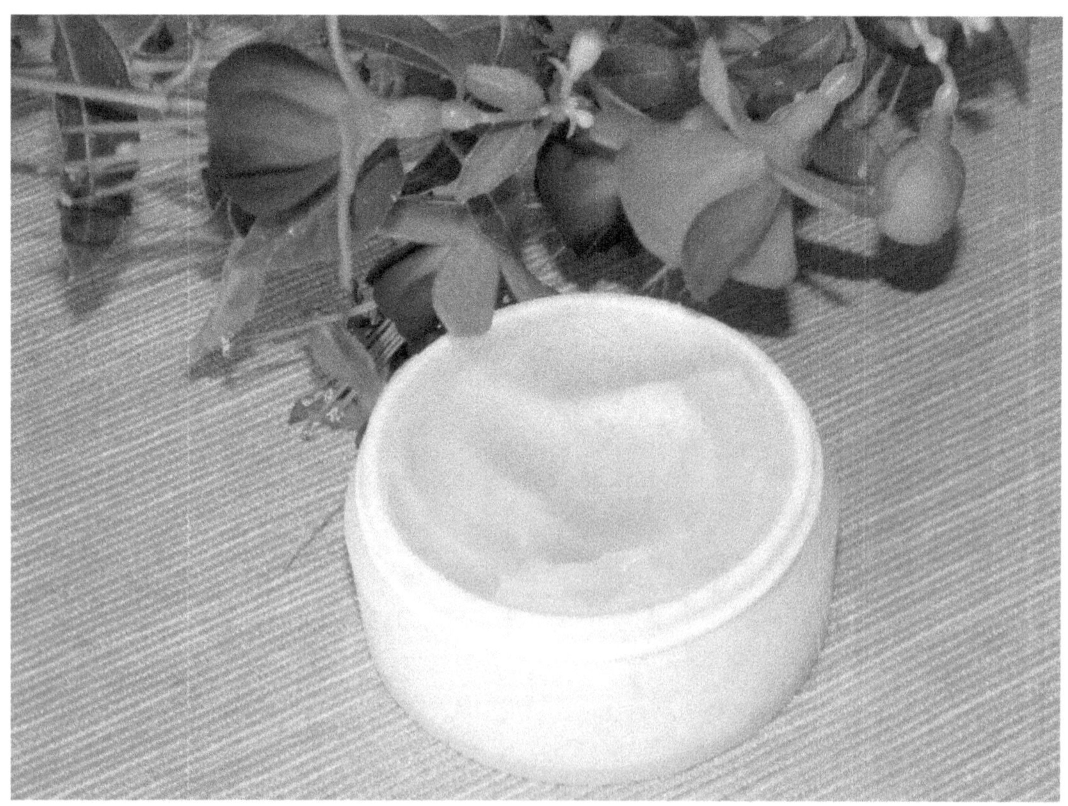

Strawberry Sunscreen

Once you start preparing your own cosmetic products, you won't be able to stop. And when it comes to sunscreen I do about 3-4 kinds/summer. I try different recipes and I use them all. If you want to do so, my advice is to prepare small quantities. You might get bored with some (like I do) and it's a shame to throw it away if you don't use it all.

There are plenty of ingredients you may use: butters (shea, cocoa, mango), oils (coconut, sweet almond, avocado, olive, sesame, red raspberry, carrot seed), beeswax (for making the sunscreen waterproof) and sun blockers (minerals like zinc oxide or titanium dioxide). Some of the oils and butter also have SPF: shea butter and coconut oil – 4-6; red raspberry oil – 25-50; carrot seed oil – 35-40; zinc oxide – about 20 (depending on how much you are using).

If you want a scented sunscreen be sure you avoid citrus essential oils. They are photo toxic and may cause skin burns.

You Will Need:

- ✓ 1/4 cup grape seed oil
- ✓ 1 tbsp beeswax pastilles
- ✓ 5 tsp zinc oxide
- ✓ 1/2 cup distilled water
- ✓ 3 tbsp aloe vera gel
- ✓ 10 drops strawberry extract

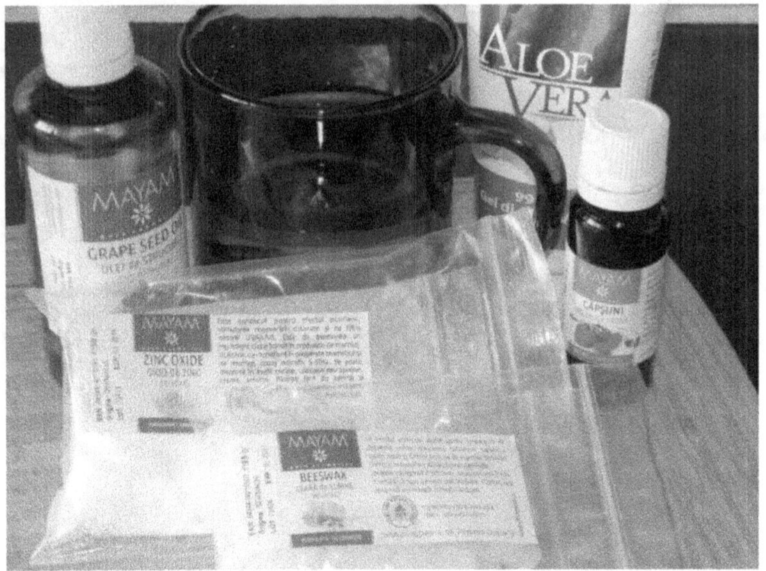

Directions:

1. Add the beeswax to a glass jar.

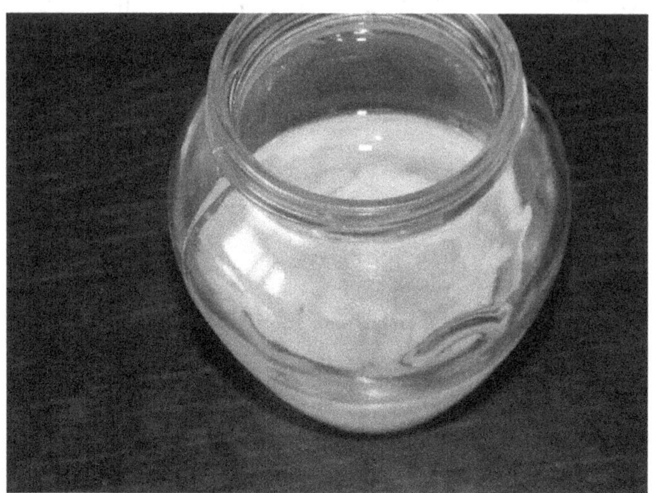

2. Melt the beeswax over low heat by placing the jar on a pan with hot water.
3. Add the oil and stir well.
4. Mix in the strawberry extract and the zinc oxide. Make sure you don't inhale the powder and that is evenly distributed.
5. Combine the distilled water and the aloe vera gel and heat them in a small pan. The mixture has to be slightly warm.
6. Add it slowly to the oil mixture and whisk well.
7. Pour everything in a dry container and let it cool.

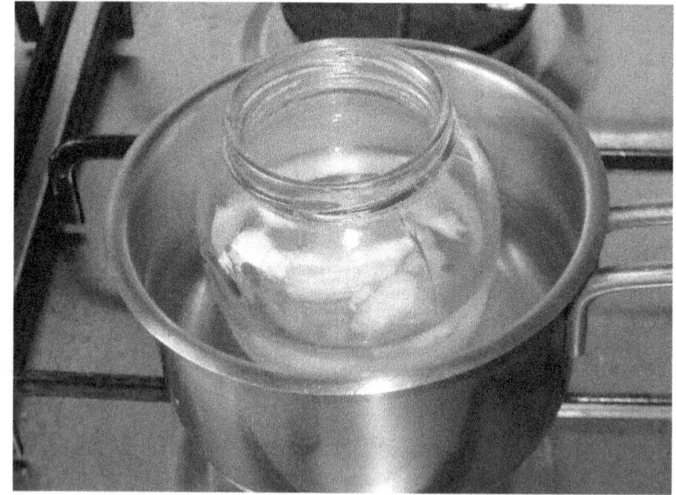

When going to the beach apply the sunscreen as often as needed, mainly after taking a bath.

Natural Bug Repellents

Generally, big bites are benign conditions. However, sometimes a simple bug bite may lead to a rash, infection or an allergic reaction. No matter your age, it is wise to try to keep bugs away from you and your family.

I included 10 insect repellent tutorials to help you and your family enjoy the outdoors.

This section will show you how to make some simple insect repellents.

For each tutorial, you get:

- A list of the ingredients you'll need to prepare the natural insect repellent
- Step by step text instructions describing how to prepare the natural insect repellent
- Supporting photos showing you how to prepare each repellent

So, let's get started making some natural insect repellent!

Castor Oil Repellent

Since she was one years old, my daughter has faced some atopic dermatitis and whenever a mosquito bit her everything started to swell. Like most mosquito bites, they're not small and they're red and inflamed. She gets what are often described as "red hard donuts" on her skin – which is typical of a mosquito bite. Within a couple of weeks, they're gone – but that's quite a while to wait when they're itchy and irritating.

So due to this persistent ailment, I began using natural ingredients and preparing my own homemade products to treat the bites. However, prevention is always better than cure and so today we're sharing this easy-to-made castor oil repellant that takes just minutes to make but is mightily effective and works wonders at keeping mosquitos at bay.

Last year I used this recipe for the first time. We went on a camping trip near a river where it was very humid and there was lots of vegetation there – a perfect environment for mosquitos.

In the evenings, between 7PM and 9PM there were so many mosquitos and other bugs around that we couldn't even talk for fear of them getting into our mouth.

But the repellent was very efficient. While we would often leave a place like this covered in bites, this time we only had a couple. I'd say that's a good result. The recipe is very easy to prepare and you may double the quantities if you need a larger amount of repellent.

The castor oil itself doesn't have a repellent effect, but it has a thicker consistency and makes a good base for the essential oil repellents work their magic.

You Will Need:

- ✓ 1 teaspoon castor oil
- ✓ 1 ½ tablespoon water
- ✓ 10 drops lemongrass essential oil
- ✓ 10 drops thyme essential oil
- ✓ 5 drops geranium essential oil

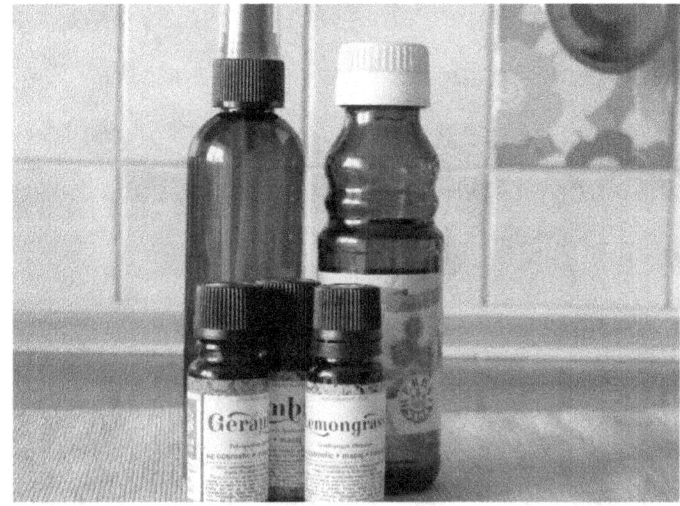

Directions:

1. Combine all the ingredients in a spray bottle.

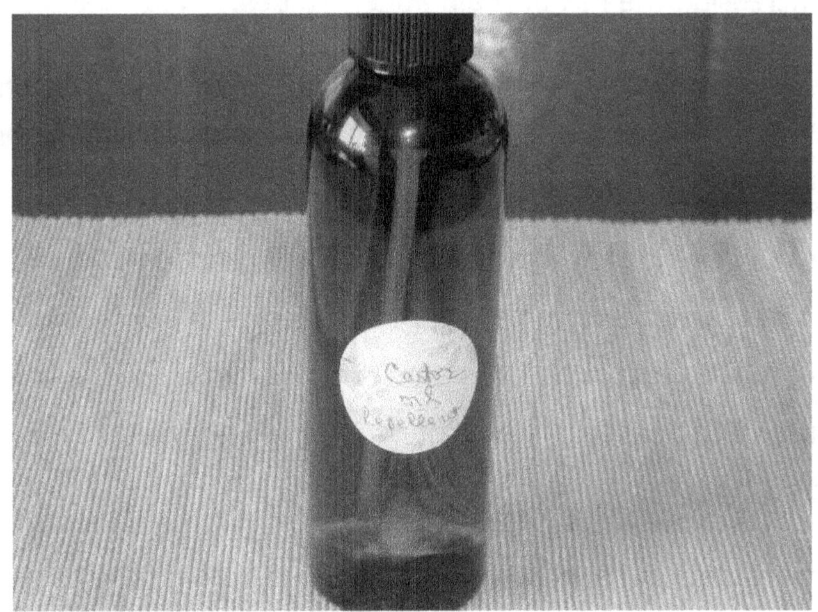

2. Shake well before each use.
3. Make sure you reapply often for getting the desired effect.

I find this natural mixture safe for my kids and we use it quite often. It is also the cheapest version I have ever tried.

Essential Oils Bug Spray – Oil Based

Citronella essential oil is well known as a very good insect repellent: it keeps away mosquitoes, spiders, ants, flies and moths. The essential oil combination from this recipe has a great smell, well, great for *us*, the insects seem to hate it and they run away from it. Which is a good thing, considering the fact that nobody likes to have them around, right?

Therefore, you should definitely use citronella in your homemade repellents. So why wouldn't you just simply run to the store to buy some product instead of preparing it yourself? Because common repellents contain DEET (N,N-Diethyl-meta-toluamide), a chemical substance proven to be neurotoxic. Adverse effects have been shown to occur even after just months or years of use. DEET, combined with other chemicals (like the ones found in repellent products or body creams, for example) becomes more dangerous, increasing the risk of brain abnormalities.

Another toxic substance which can be found on the ingredients list of common repellents is permethrin from the pyrethroid family. It may cause tremors, loss of coordination, increased temperature, aggressive behavior, inability to learn or eat, agitation. It is carcinogenic (it is directly linked to cancer) and leads to the formation of lung tumors in females and liver tumors in both sexes. It is involved in chromosomal abnormalities and impedes the proper functioning of the immune system. It also causes damages to the environment by killing bees, fish and poultry and cats. Quite scary, right?

And, since the homemade repellents are so easy to prepare and also healthy (as they contain only natural ingredients) I strongly suggest you should try this recipe at home.

You Will Need:

- ✓ 10 drops citronella essential oil
- ✓ 10 drops tea tree oil
- ✓ 10 drops lemongrass oil
- ✓ 5 drops lemon essential oil
- ✓ 5 drops cedar essential oil
- ✓ 2 oz sweet almond oil

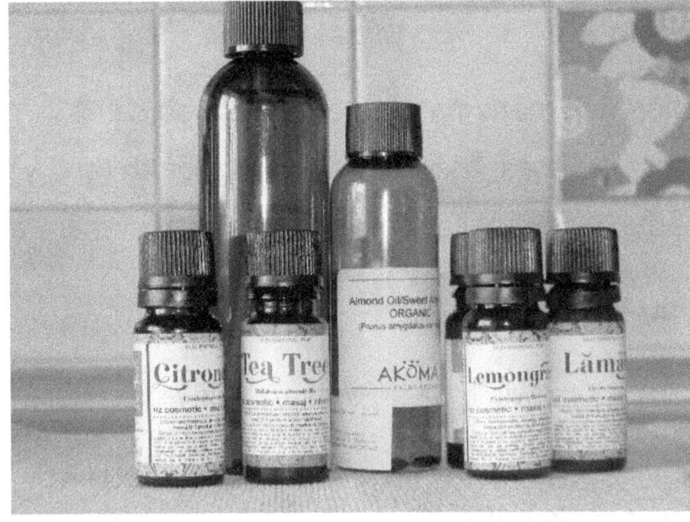

Directions:

1. Take a spray recipient and combine all the ingredients.
2. Shake well before each use, so everything is well distributed.

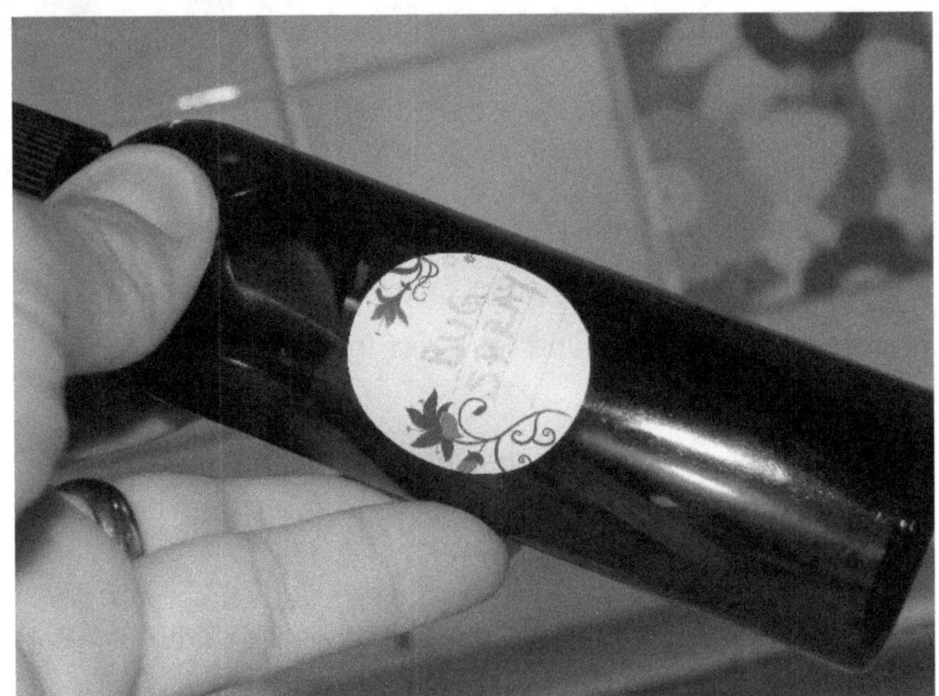

This mixture is suitable for children 2+ years old.

Essential Oils Bug Spray – Water Based

There are many natural repellents you can try. You should stay away from the chemical ones, they may put your health (and your children's health) at risk. The homemade repellents are very easy to prepare and they won't harm you at all.

You Will Need:

- ✓ 2 oz witch hazel/vodka/apple cider vinegar
- ✓ 2 oz water
- ✓ 10 drops citronella essential oil
- ✓ 10 drops tea tree oil
- ✓ 10 drops lemongrass essential oil
- ✓ 5 drops lemon essential oil
- ✓ 5 drops cedar essential oil
- ✓ ¼ teaspoon castile/baby soap

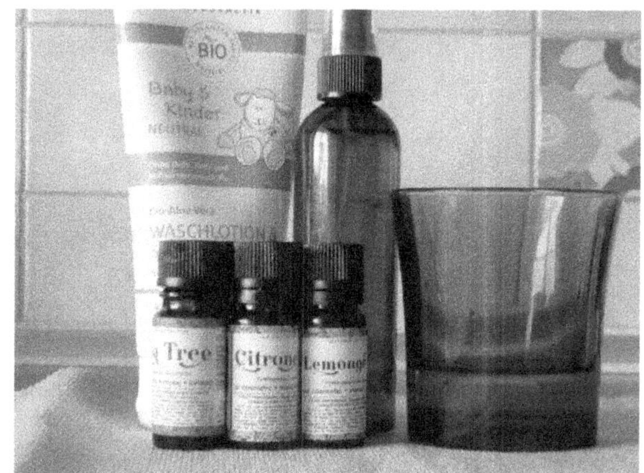

Directions:

1. I used apple cider vinegar, so I mix it with all the essential oils.
2. Then you should add the castile/baby soap. Don't shake at this point so the essential oils disperse in the liquid. Just let it rest for 5 minutes.
3. After that shake the container well.
4. Mix in the water and shake again. You should do this each time before you use the spray.

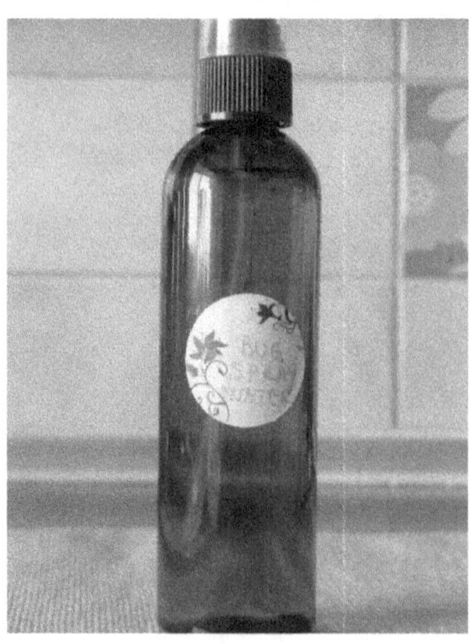

This mixture is suitable for children 2+ years old. Smaller children may not tolerate the essential oils combination so well.

Remember that those fragrances are very powerful compounds that may harm a sensitive skin even if they are all-natural. Make sure you use essential oils that are suitable for your child's age.

Insect Repellent

There are many insects that could spoil a long planned camping trip, a romantic evening or even a nice play in the park.

The shelves of the stores are filled with repellents that are "good" for everyone, including babies and children.

But when you take a closer look you may find that they contain a substance called DEET which:

- has been associated with seizures followed by even death in some cases;
- is prohibited in many countries. Where allowed, it is recommended not to use in children under two years (or other sources under 6 years), nor by pregnant women. The rest should apply maximum once a day, with local washing after the repellent effect is no longer wanted. I hope that all commercial anti-mosquito solutions for children have this information presented on the label so that parents can make an informed choice.
- the substance was patented by US military's in the Gulf War.

It is better to use a natural insect repellent which you can easily make at home...

You Will Need:

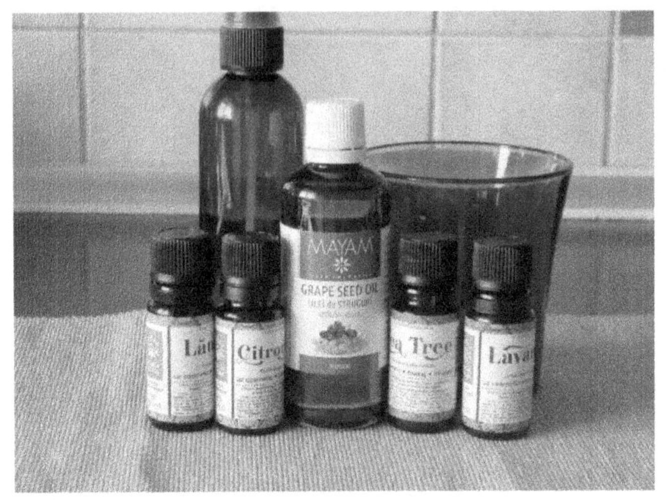

- ✓ 1 oz grape seed oil
- ✓ 1 oz vodka/apple cider vinegar
- ✓ 15 drops citronella essential oil
- ✓ 10 drops lavender essential oil
- ✓ 10 drops lemon essential oil
- ✓ 5 drops tea tree essential oil

Directions:

1. Use a glass recipient to combine all the ingredients.
2. Shake so that they are well distributed.
3. Spray every time is necessary, usually every 90-120 minutes.

You shouldn't expect a natural repellent to last as long as a chemical one.

The smell of the essential oils will be stronger in the beginning, but it will start to fade as the time passes.

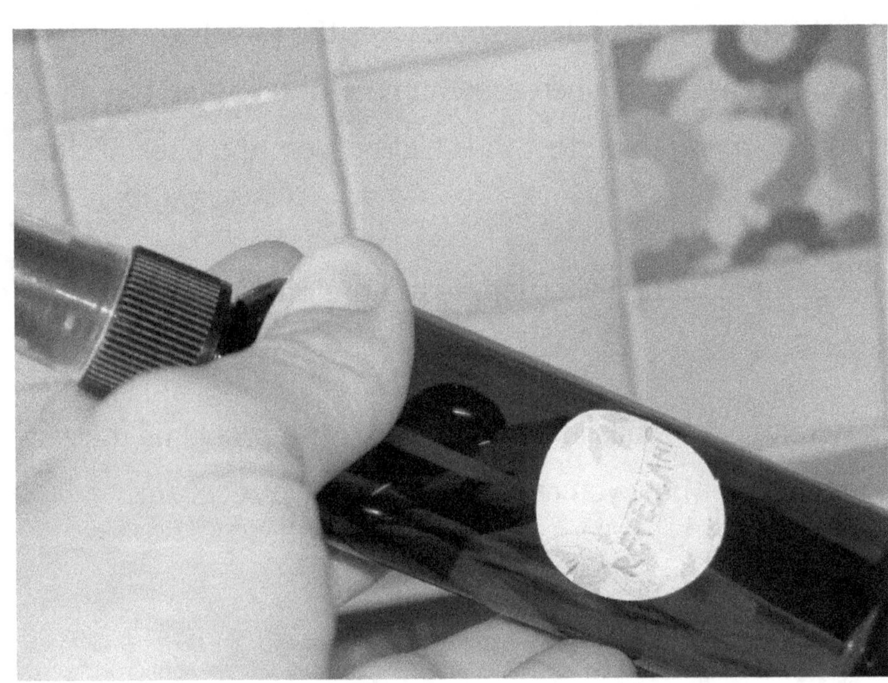

So, keep the spray close to you and use it when you see the insects come back. The natural mixture will keep them away for certain and they won't bother you anymore.

The repellent is suitable for children 2+ years.

Ticks and mosquitoes are small, but they can spread very dangerous diseases. Prevention is the first step for the fight against these insects as we cannot spend all summer dressed in long pants, socks and boots.

Repellents are a great solution. Most of the trade ones are based on chemicals and some of them are quite dangerous. Over the past few years parents especially are very worried about the increased number of ticks and the diseases they can spread. Everyone is trying to protect the children from the bites of those tiny yet dangerous insects.

However more natural alternatives are preferred to those based on permethrin, for example.

Fortunately, nature has left solutions to these problems that anyone can afford. Here is an idea about how you can create your own repellent.

You Will Need:

- ✓ white wine vinegar
- ✓ dried lavender flowers

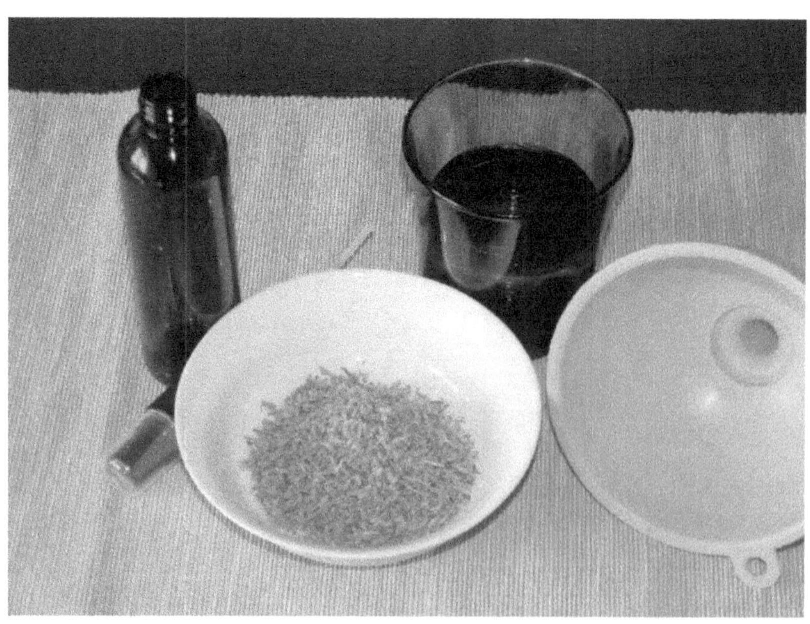

Directions:

1. You will need a 3 oz bottle spray.
2. Use a funnel to place the dried lavender flowers in the bottle. The flowers should reach almost to the top.

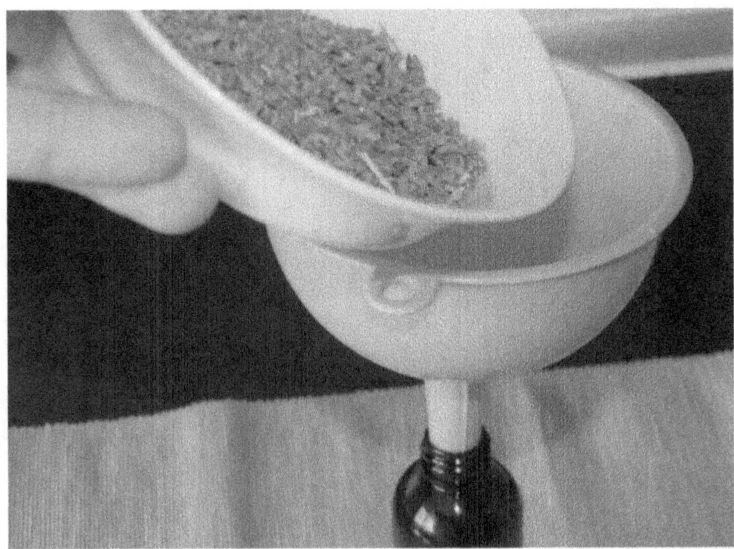

3. Pour the white wine vinegar to fill in the bottle.

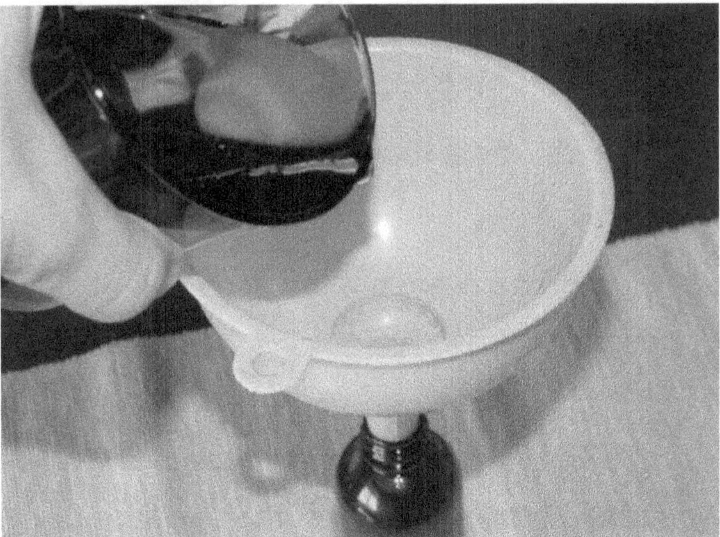

4. You should leave the mixture to infuse for at least one week. Remember to shake daily for the ingredients to mix well.
5. After the infusion period is done, strain the liquid.
6. Use as an insect repellent every time you need it.

7. This mixture can also be used for insect bites, it relieves the itchiness or the pain.

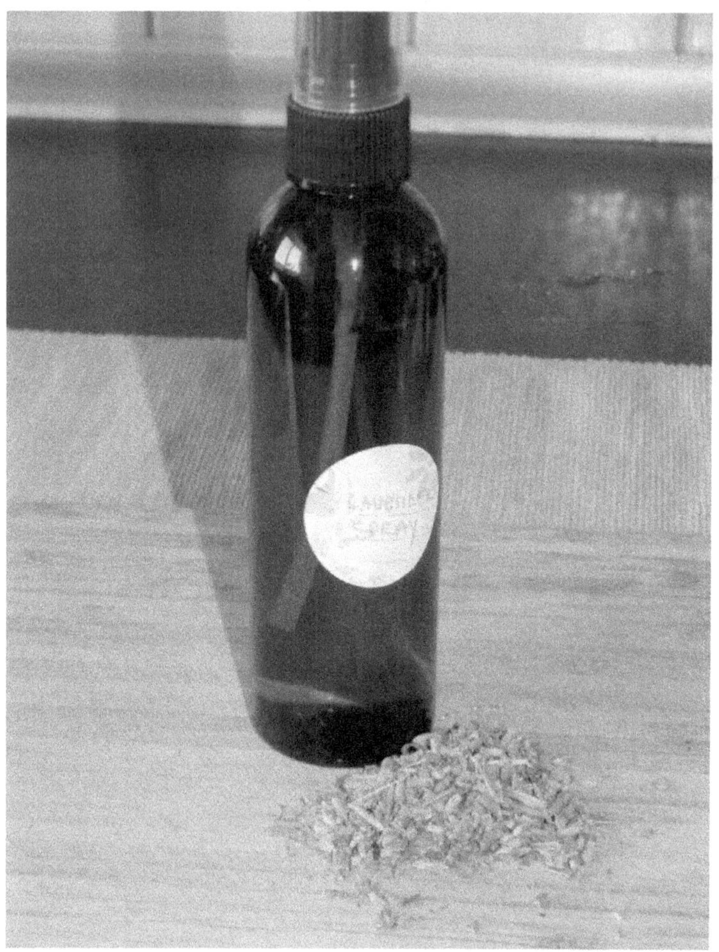

This combination has a distinctive smell and insects are not very fond of it. It works really well against mosquitoes, ticks, bugs and fleas.

You may use it for children 2+ years old. The babies' skin is very sensitive, and you must pay attention to everything you use with them. First, test the repellent: apply to a very small area and watch it for at least 24 hours. If there are no signs of allergy or irritation continue the use.

Natural Fly Spray

Flies are insects of the Diptera order (derived from the Greek term, di = two and pteron = wing), possessing only one pair of wings on the median thorax and a pair of sheath. The Housefly is one of the most popular insects. Diptera order is a general order, including an estimated number of over 240,000 different varieties of insect species, although only about half of them have been studied and described (about 120,000 species) according to the estimates.

Most flies feed on organic matter even with that in undergoing decomposition. Flies sit on anything and basically eat anything, which means they're dirty and not something you want flying around your home.

To prevent flies from coming next to your home biodegradable garbage should be discarded regularly and as quickly as possible.

Potential hatching places, such as manure and compost should be placed away from home. To keep the flies outside of your house you should install nets on the windows and the balcony doors.

A natural repellent can also help you with the flies. Here's how to make one.

You Will Need:

- ✓ 20 drops tea tree essential oil
- ✓ 20 drops thyme essential oil
- ✓ 20 drops lavender essential oil
- ✓ 1-quart apple cider vinegar

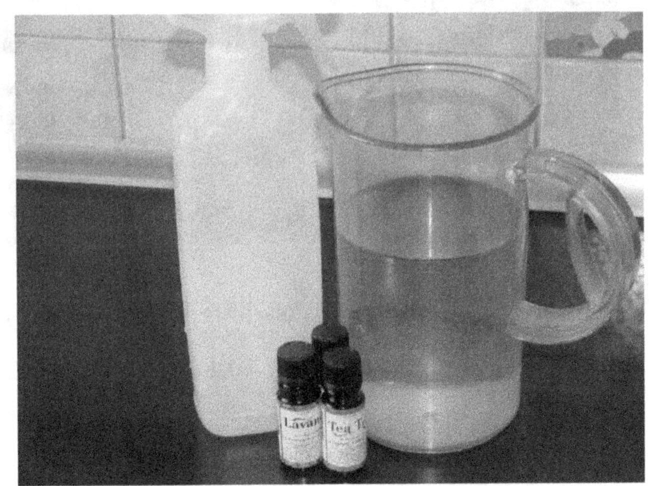

Directions:

1. Place all the ingredients in a spray bottle.
2. Shake well before each use.

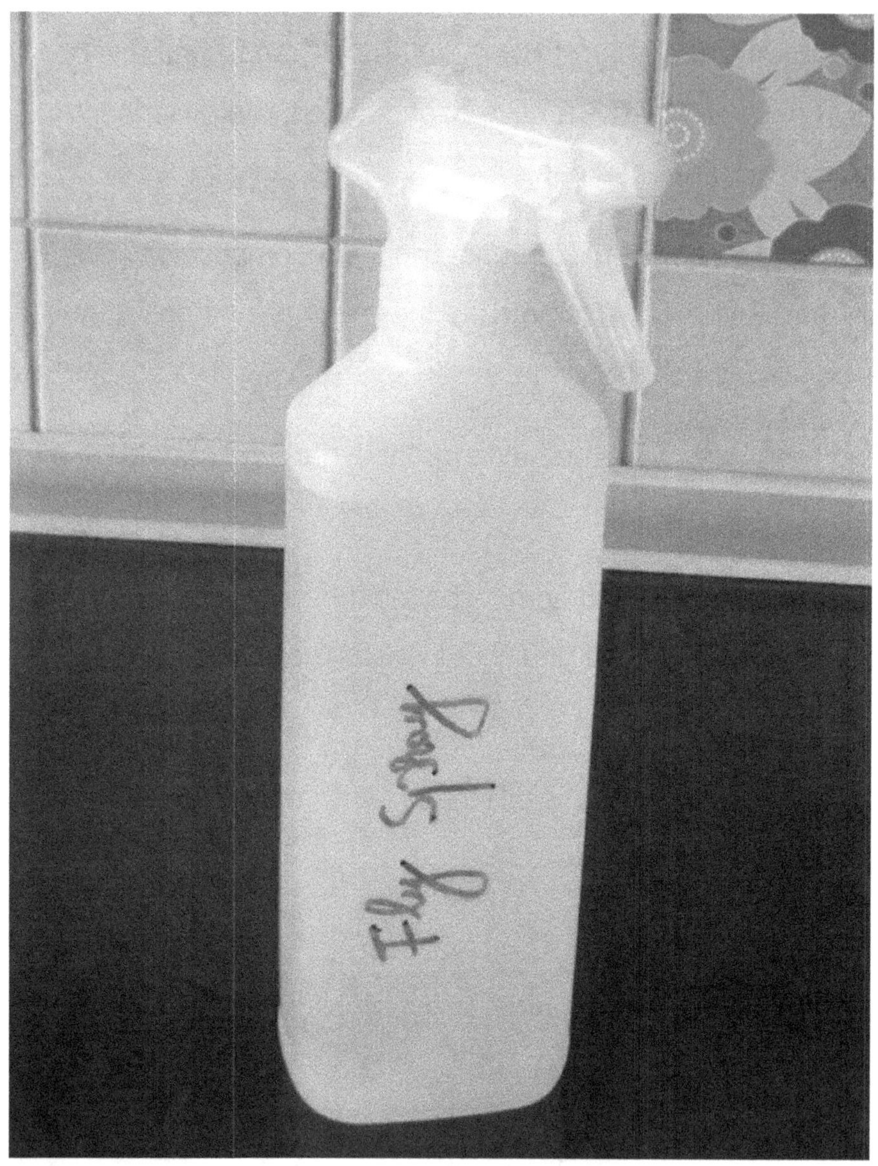

Apply whenever you see those flies prowl. The spray has a strong smell and the insects don't like it, so they try to keep away. This is a really good choice for you and your family. The repellent is all-natural and brings no harm to human health.

Natural Mosquito Spray

Mosquitoes have complex methods of screening potential "hosts" and, depending on their type, they react to different stimuli. Most mosquitoes are active at dusk and when it's getting darker but there are certain species that seek "hosts" during the whole day.

You can avoid their bites either by making sure you do not draw them in any way, either directing them to other areas or using specific repellents.

Here's what activities and objects can attract more mosquitoes (it is good to know these things so you can avoid them):

- Dark clothes because most mosquitoes use their eyes to detect the hosts. Dark objects and foliage are the first to enter their spotlight
- Carbon dioxide – you eliminate more carbon dioxide when you are hot or sweating. Equally appealing to mosquitoes can be lighted candles or other sources of ignition
- Lactic acid - eliminated after exercising or ingestion of certain foods (products with high salt or potassium)
- Floral or fruity fragrances that can be found in perfumes, hair products and sunscreens (they can be found in fabric softener too)
- The body temperature is also a trigger for mosquitoes, some species are attracted to slightly colder temperature of the extremities
- Moisture - mosquitoes are attracted to sweat because of the chemicals it contains and of the humidity created around the body; even small amounts of water can attract these insects accounting them as possible breeding locations

To Make A Natural Mosquito Spray, You Will Need:

- ✓ Distilled water
- ✓ 10 drops geranium essential oil
- ✓ 30 drops tea tree essential oil
- ✓ 1 tablespoon glycerin
- ✓ 1/2 teaspoon vanilla extract

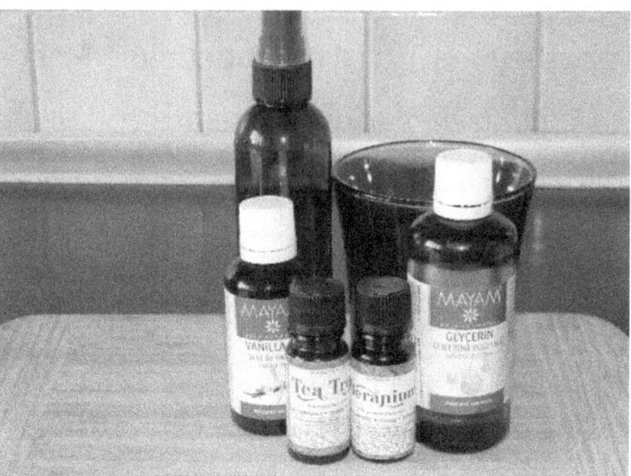

Directions:

1. Combine the essential oils and the vanilla extract.
2. Add the vegetable glycerin.
3. Fill a 3 oz bottle with water and shake well before use.

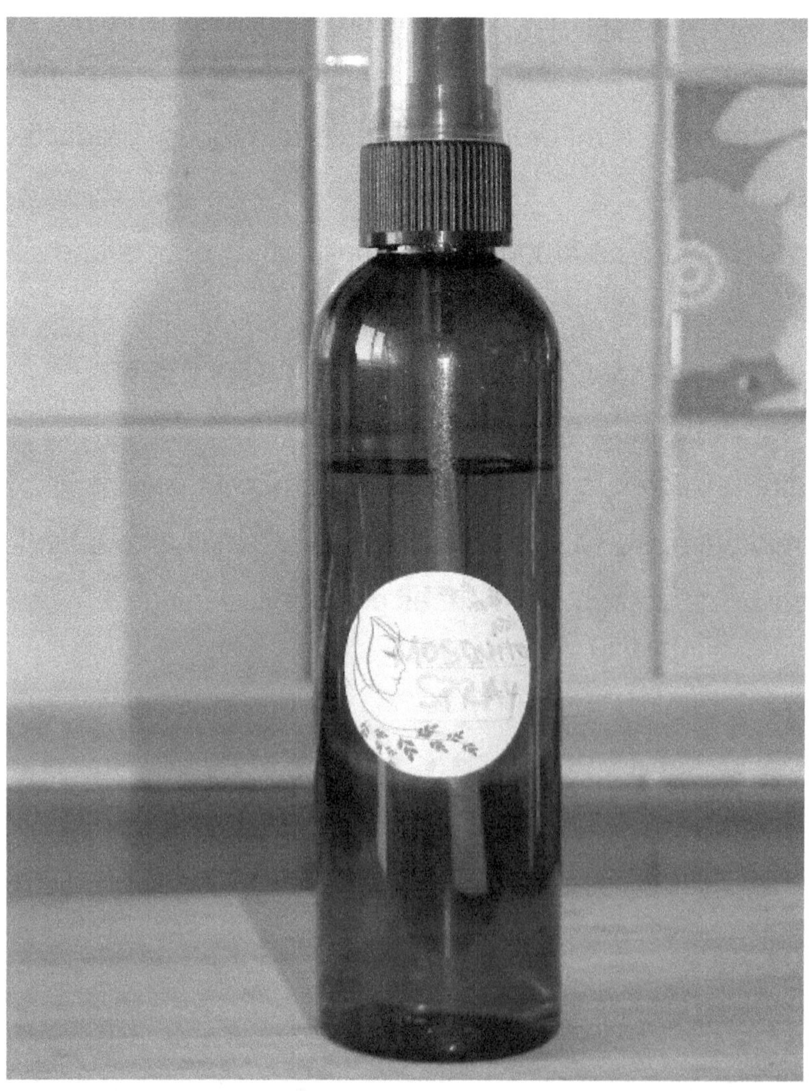

Neem Oil Repellent

In ancient Vedic culture, neem tree is referred to as "Sarva Roga Nirvarini" - capable of curing every disease and every illness. Neem has been used in India for thousands of years and is widely used in Ayurveda for its power to fight the diseases.

Every part of the tree - branches, leaves, bark, fruits, flowers and roots are extremely beneficial because they contain a special compound called azadirachtin which is giving neem its anti-bacterial, anti-fungal and anti-parasitic effects. Neem is extremely beneficial in treating various infections and it empowers the immune system. Apart from a number of health benefits, it is also used in a variety of household products. Neem is safe to use and does not lead to side effects.

Neem oil is a vegetable oil extracted from the fruits and seeds of the neem tree. Its color ranges from light brown to dark brown depending on the extraction method. It is a very bitter-tasting oil, mainly due to triglycerides and triterpene compounds. This oil is used for many purposes. Neem oil contains fatty acids such as oleic acid and linoleic acid, which are beneficial to the skin.

It also smells extremely bad, but if you combine it with some flavored essential oils you won't be able to feel the smell anymore.

You Will Need:

- ✓ 10 drops neem oil
- ✓ 15 drops geranium essential oil
- ✓ 15 drops lavender essential oil
- ✓ 15 drops lemon essential oil
- ✓ 2 oz jojoba/coconut oil

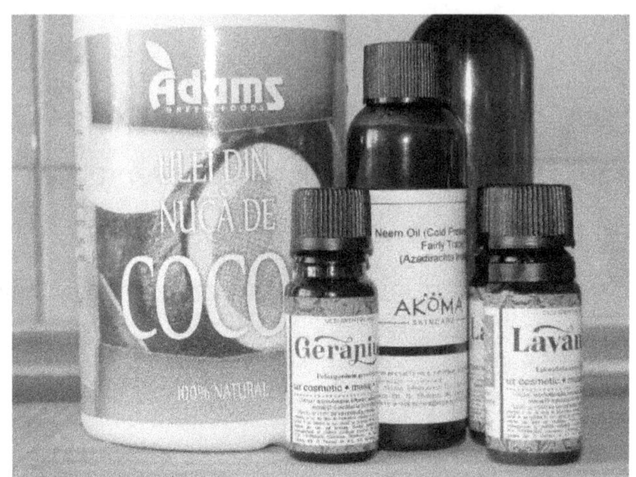

Directions:

1. Combine all the ingredients and mix well.
2. Store in a spray bottle and use whenever necessary.

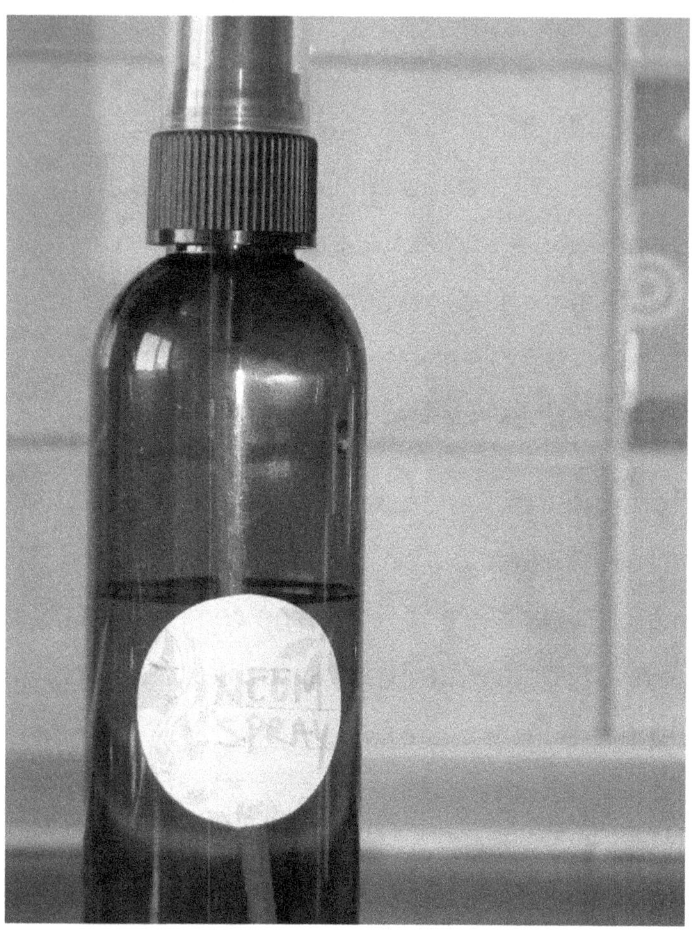

As you see, homemade repellents are quite easy to prepare. You only need a carrier oil (like jojoba, coconut, sunflower or even olive oil) and a mix of essential oils that will keep the insects away. Those nasty invaders hate the smell of lavender, for example, not to mention the neem one so they will go away from you and your family.

Why don't we use commercially available repellents in our house, on our skin or the skin of our babies?

Considering how toxic they are I feel bad that I use them on my dogs and that I don't find some time to create a natural one for them too. But I definitely could not knowingly use those common repellents on my children's skin.

I advise you to carefully read the ingredients' lists, even the ones from the products that are "especially created for children". All of them contain DEET (N, N-Diethyl-meta-toluamide).

This substance:

- is a carcinogen;
- it destroys the hormonal system;
- it is neurotoxic;
- affects the olfactory system;
- it is causing insomnia;
- affects cognitive functions;
- irritates eyes and skin;
- causes memory loss, headaches, weakness, fatigue, muscle and wrists pain or nausea;
- inhibits the central nervous system, especially in relation to the muscular system, causing neuromuscular paralysis and often death by asphyxiation.

I really don't like how all these sound. Kind of creepy! I really cannot picture myself putting something like this on my kids. So, I prepared my own repellent which is completely natural and safe.

You Will Need:

- ✓ 15 drops patchouli essential oil
- ✓ 15 drops cedar essential oil
- ✓ 10 drops geranium essential oil
- ✓ 4 oz grape seed oil

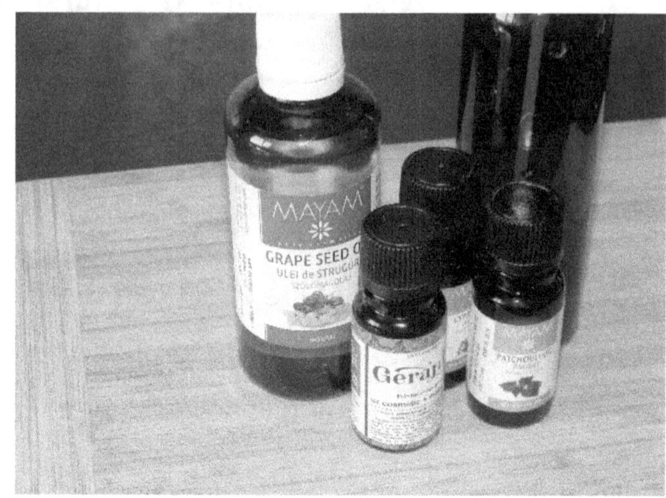

Directions:

1. Find a spray bottle or a regular one.
2. Place all the ingredients inside and mix well.
3. Shake before each use.

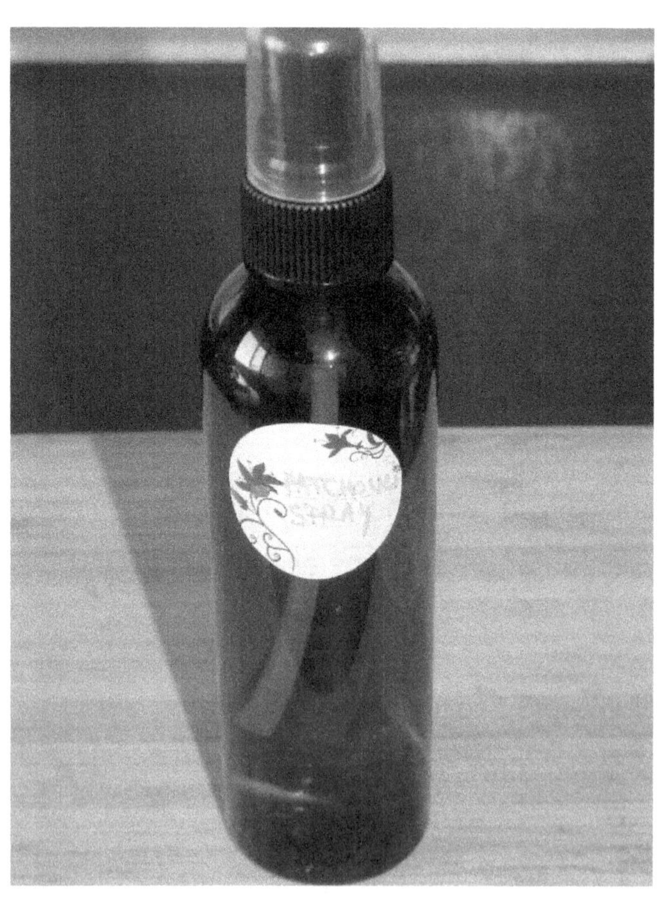

This spray will successfully keep away all the insects that would want to spoil your evening or even your holiday. You will be able to have a wonderful camping trip together with your family, with no uninvited guests.

This repellent is suitable for children 2+ years old.

Peppermint Spray

The summer is here and along with it a lot of visitors are coming: ants, mosquitoes, spiders, bugs, ticks and so on. They all rush into your house, your kitchen and even your bedroom. And this is no good at all.

I really don't like killing them. I have a deep respect for all living beings. If they don't put me or my family in danger, I prefer leaving them alone. But they should do the same for me!

I used to buy all kind of repellents from the store. Besides the chemicals listed as ingredients, they do smell awful. I hate that smell. It really irritates me, and I began to have headaches so I decided to stop buying them.

But that didn't solve my insect problem at all, as the bugs kept coming. I had to do something to chase them away for keeping my mental sanity. I remembered the essential oils. And if they are really effective with the mosquitoes, they might as well work with the other pests, right?

One of the most powerful essential oils is peppermint. The bugs dislike the strong smell so much that they don't want to be in a place with such flavor. They stay far away and that's what they *should* do.

You Will Need:

- ✓ 1 tablespoon vegetable glycerin
- ✓ Water
- ✓ 20 drops peppermint essential oil

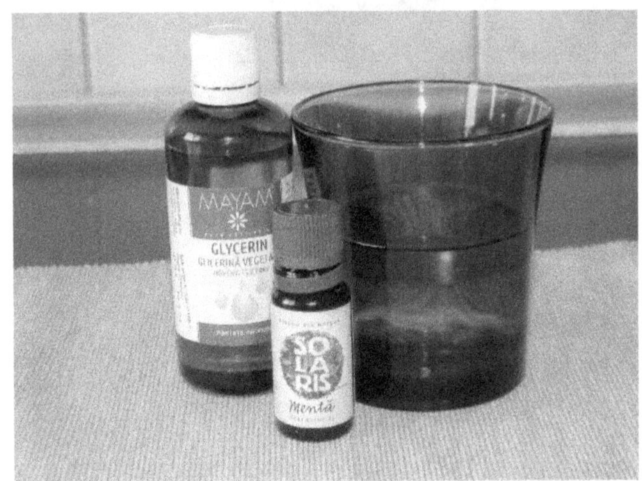

Directions:

1. Put the essential oil in the spray recipient you are using.
2. Add the glycerin and mix well.
3. Fill a 2 oz bottle with water and shake before each use.

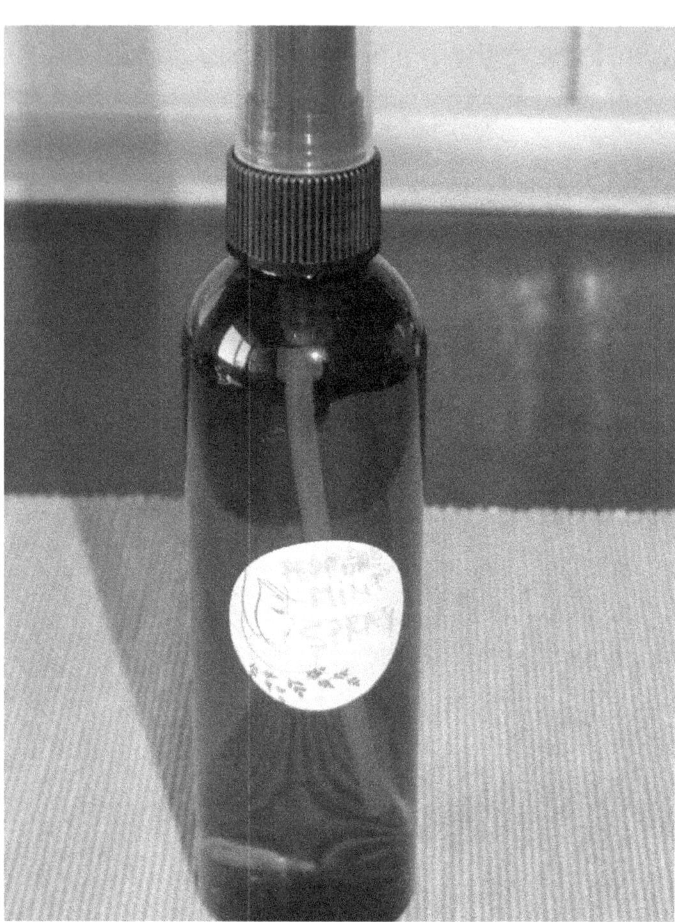

2+

This spray will successfully keep away all the insects that would want to spoil your evening or even your holiday. You will be able to have a wonderful camping trip together with your family, with no uninvited guests.

This repellent is suitable for children

Everyone knows that plants are good because they give us oxygen and get rid of carbon dioxide. It is less commonly known that some house plants filter toxins out of the air in our homes and places of work. They are so effective that NASA prefers them over high-tech air purifying devices for space stations. Once you have read up on these amazing plants you might not be able to resist finding one for yourself.

NASA Clean Air Study

NASA did a study called "Interior Landscape Plants for Indoor Air Pollution Abatement." Around the 1970s it became apparent that sealing buildings shut, for improved efficiency of heating and air conditioning, was making residents and workers sick. Newly created synthetic building materials started off-gassing into the indoor air, which meant that the chemicals were evaporating into the air and stayed there because of a lack of airflow. The air was being filled with Volatile Organic Compounds (VOCs) such as formaldehyde, benzene and trichloroethylene.

It was the building materials, the furniture and often cleaning products that were causing massive indoor air pollution with hundreds of volatile organics, which do damage on their own and create even more pollution as they react with each other.

Governments then enforced stricter regulations on the amounts of VOCs in products.

NASA did a study on how house plants (and their soil microorganisms) might clean up indoor air pollution, hoping to improve the air in their space stations.

The NASA Clean Air Study was run in collaboration with the Associated Landscape Contractors of America in 1989. NASA was looking for a way to clean the indoor air of space stations and decided to test out house plants. Scientists were already aware that indoor plants absorb carbon dioxide and produce oxygen, but they wanted to know if plants could get rid of toxins too.

The study tested house plants and the 5 most common VOCs, xylene, benzene, trichloroethylene, formaldehyde, trichloroethylene, toluene and they also tested ammonia. The heaviest of hitters of the plants were the Peace Lilly and the Florists Chrysanthemum as they filtered out all 5 VOCs tested. The Variegated Snake Plant also stands out in that it is the hardest to kill and can handle low light and neglectful owners.

Volatile Organic Compounds

NASA found that some house plants are effective at purifying the air of Volatile Organic Compounds (VOCs). VOCs are chemicals that are releasing vapors from materials, a process called off-gassing, into the air.

Lots of odors are VOCs. Most VOCs are extremely bad for human health. The results showed that many house plants do naturally clean the air in an enclosed space, such as a home or an office space. Some plants even absorb mold, allergens and air-born fecal matter.

VOC side effects vary. Medical professionals are concerned that, although you may feel no immediate symptoms, these toxic chemicals might be damaging your health in ways you're not even aware of. Also, VOCs refer to many different chemicals. Each chemical has its own side effects. Health problems can also depend on how concentrated the VOCs are, the length of time you are exposed and how often you are exposed.

VOCs affect everyone nowadays as they are in so many products we use regularly. VOCs are particularly harmful to babies, children, expecting mothers and the elderly. People with conditions such as Fibromyalgia and Chronic Fatigue Syndrome are highly sensitive to most non-organic compounds.

Sick Building Syndrome

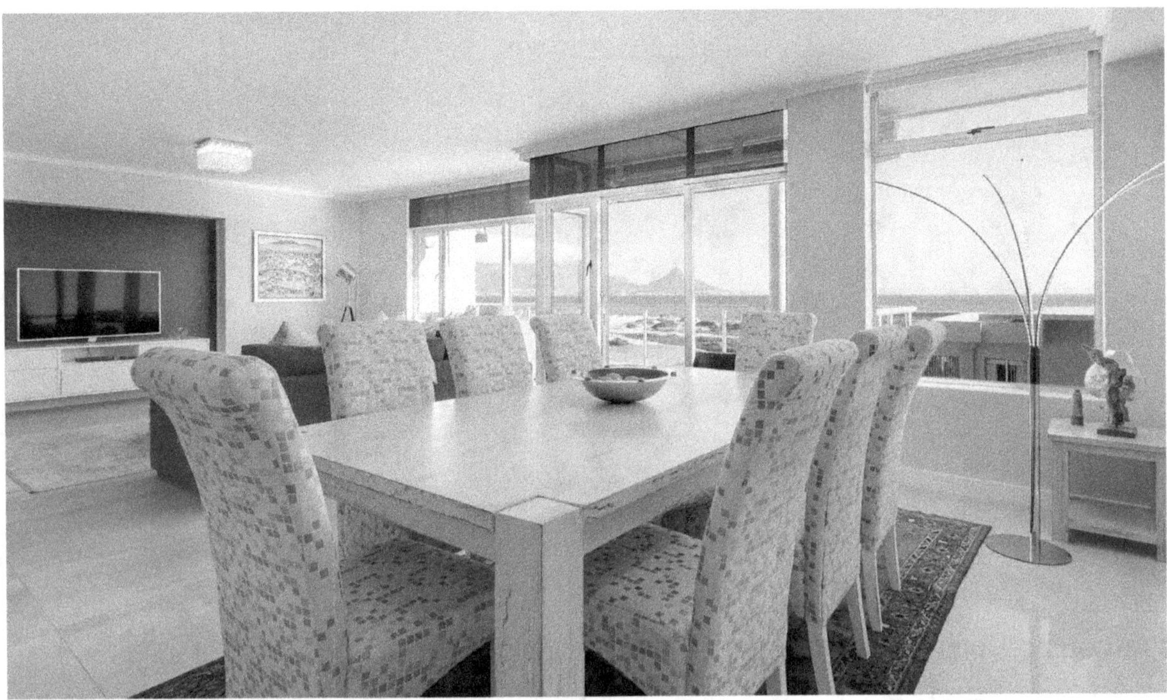

Modern buildings have extremely efficient heating and air-conditioning and there is not much airflow. Toxins build up and never get circulated out of an open window. Sick building syndrome happens when people get sick for unexplained reasons.

The condition gets worse the more time they spend in the building and sometimes gets better when they are away from the building. Some immediate symptoms include headaches, respiratory problems, fatigue, nausea, and dizziness. Long-term exposure can cause cancer and other debilitating diseases.

To cut down on exposer to VOCs, the first and easiest step is to switch to organic cleaning products. After that try to store paint, paint strippers, varnish, glue, carpet shampoo, pesticides, and all other chemicals in the garage or other structure outside the home.

Another major change is to buy organic mattresses, especially crib mattresses and mattresses for children. The VOCs noxious fumes from mattresses are surrounding young ones as they sleep for long stretches of time. Schedule a day of the week where you air out the house.

Off-gassing

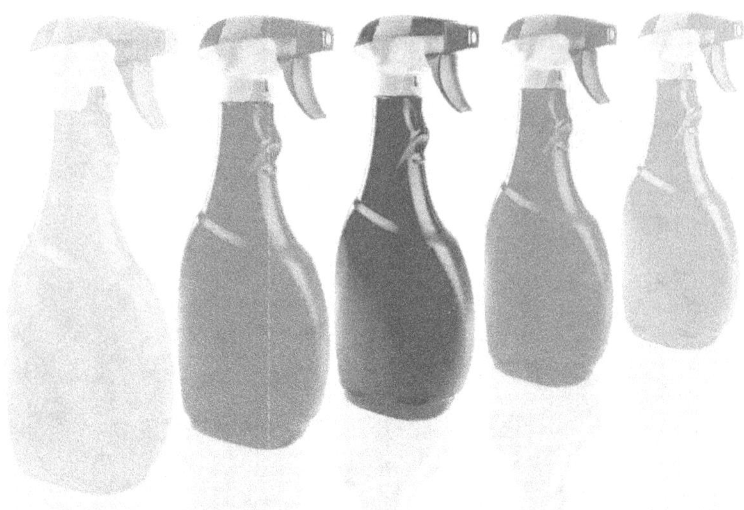

The most famous off-gassing is 'new car smell'. Basically, it is the emission of chemicals off the materials a product was made of. They are noxious gasses. The off-gassing from a product can carry on for years after purchase, ruining the air quality in your home.

Household products have the worst off-gassing. Because these products are used indoors, the noxious fumes typically stay in the indoor environment. Products such as paint, varnish, pesticides, disinfecting and cleaning products are the most toxic. Pieces of furniture fresh from the factory are also big offenders.

Benzene

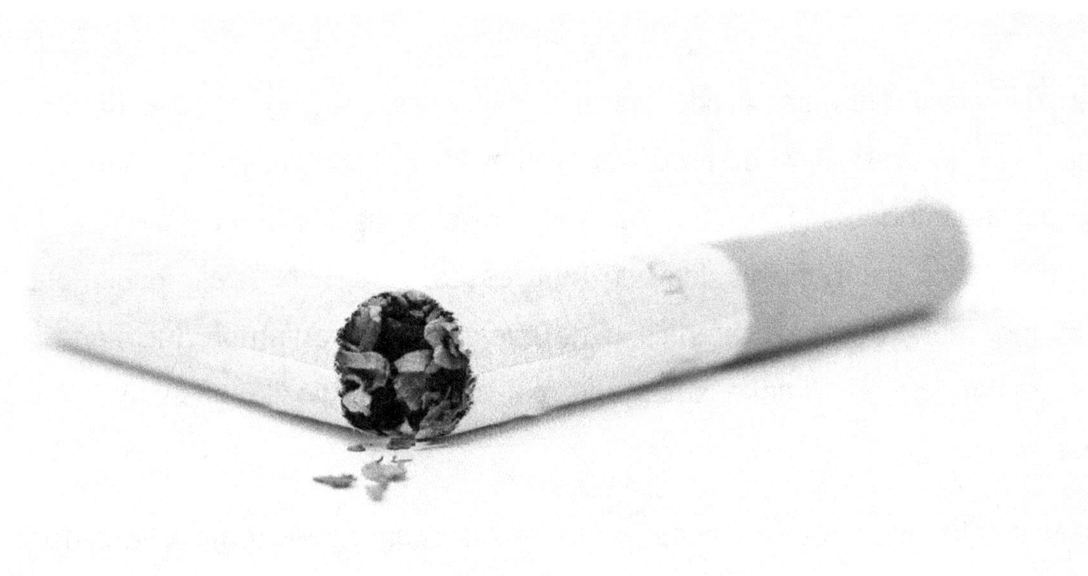

Benzene is a well-known human carcinogen. It is heavier than air so it sinks down low and tends to stay there; making is especially dangerous for children. It is used to make nylon fibres, plastics, rubbers, detergents, drugs and pesticides. Exposure to Benzene causes cancer, bone marrow failure, acute leukemia and cardiovascular disease. In 1948 the American Petroleum Institute made the statement that there was absolutely no safe expose level for benzene. Even the smallest amounts are dangerous.

Indoor areas that contain benzene are enclosed spaces that contain gasoline, glues, solvents, paints, and art supplies and cigarette smoke

Levels of benzene are higher in homes that are close to gas stations and homes that have attached garages.

Chronic and regular exposure to benzene causes acute myeloid leukaemia and childhood leukemia along with other forms of cancer.

Short-term side effects to breathing in benzene are similar to getting "high" such as; dizziness, confusion and unconsciousness.

Formaldehyde

Formaldehyde is found in many products that are indoors, causing massive indoor air pollution. It is in pressed-wood products such as MDF, plywood and particleboard; meaning it is in furniture such as bookshelves, kitchen cabinets, desks and beds. It's also in paint, plastic, leather, mattresses, glue, adhesives, insulation, resins, clothing, many building materials, synthetic fabrics, cleaning products and cosmetics. It is in cigarette smoke, smog and fuel-burning items like gas stoves, and space heaters.

Formaldehyde is known to cause cancer; namely brain cancer, leukemia and cancer of the nasal sinuses among other types. It might also trigger childhood asthma.

Formaldehyde in the indoor air, at levels higher than 0.1 parts per million, can cause watery eyes, coughing, nausea and skin problems. Indoor air often contains more formaldehyde than outdoor air.

Formaldehyde in cosmetics and lotions can cause an allergic reaction of the skin but it also off-gasses from products into the air.

Trichloroethylene

Trichloroethylene (TCE) is used primarily as an industrial solvent but is in household products as well, such as; paint removers, adhesives, spot removers and rug-cleaning fluids. It is the most common contaminate in groundwater. TCE can enter a home through contaminated water and then off-gasses into the air. According to the Agency for Toxic Substances and Disease Registry there is some Trichloroethylene in 9% to 34% of drinking water in the United States and those numbers are continuing to rise.

Human and animal studies have proven that TCE causes cancer such as kidney, cervix and liver. According to the Environmental Protection Agency, short term and long-term exposure causes dizziness, euphoria, headaches, confusion and weakness.

Xylene

Xylene is a cause for concern because it is in so many common products. It is sometimes in paints, adhesives, varnishes, gasoline, rubber, cement, printing, leathers, pesticides, insecticides, aerosol paints, agricultural chemicals, caulking, epoxy adhesives, floor polishes, herbicides, markers, pet flea and tick products and shoe polish. Xylene vapour is heavier than air and may settle in to lower areas.

Symptoms of exposure are headaches, respiratory problems, central nervous system problems, confusion, dizziness and balance problems. Long-term exposure can cause problems with the central nervous system such as dizziness, headaches, tremors, and cardiovascular problems. Exposure can also cause impaired gait (changes in walking), rapid breathing, and loss of consciousness, coma and death. A single, minor exposure to xylene is not likely to cause long-term effects. Xylene is not known to cause cancer.

Xylene sniffing has been used as a way to get high and can cause heart, kidney, brain and muscle damage.

Toluene

Toluene is found in fingernail polish, adhesives, paint, paint thinners, rubber, lacquers and leathers. It is also in gasoline, which makes it more likely to be in homes near high traffic areas.

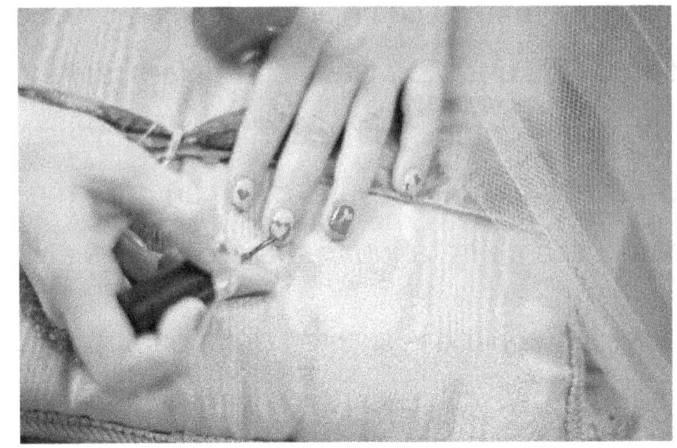

Toluene causes indoor air pollution where paint thinners or solvents are used or where smoking is allowed.

Toluene enters ground water at landfills and underground storage tanks can leak and contaminate the soil.

The majority of toluene you have ingested leaves your body within a day. With daily exposure a small amount will accumulate in fat tissue. Low doses may cause an effect on the brain and nerves. Low doses can cause temporary problems like dizziness, headaches or unconsciousness.

More serious effects come with abusing (huffing) toluene for its euphoric effects. Exposure may also cause liver and kidney damage. Moderate, day-to-day, exposure can cause tiredness, weakness and memory loss. Children are exposed to toluene by family use of glues, adhesives or cleaning solvents. Toluene is heavier than air and so sinks down to children's height.

Reduce your risk of exposure by only using toluene-containing products by using them in well-ventilated areas. Children and adolescents have used toluene-containing products to get high and so these products should be properly sealed and stored to discourage this behaviour.

Ammonia

Ammonia is not a Volatile Organic Compound but NASA tested it during the Clean Air Study.

Ammonia is in many commercial cleaning products as well as many pharmaceutical products. It is used to manufacture plastics, fabrics, dyes, pesticides and other products. It is common in household and industrial cleaning products. In its concentrated form it is caustic and can burn the skin. Even in small concentrations ammonia can be irritating to the eyes, lungs and skin.

Because ammonia has such a strong odour, you will typically smell it before it will do you harm. However, people will asthma and chemical sensitivities, might be affected by low levels of ammonia. Ammonia exposure does not cause cancer.

Combing the information we have today on VOCS, off-gassing, and Sick Building Syndrome is inspiring enough to justify spending a little money on some plants. The first thing to consider is where you have the room for a plant where it will have the appropriate amount of sunlight.

12 Air Cleansing Plant to Have in Your Home and Office

Aloe Vera

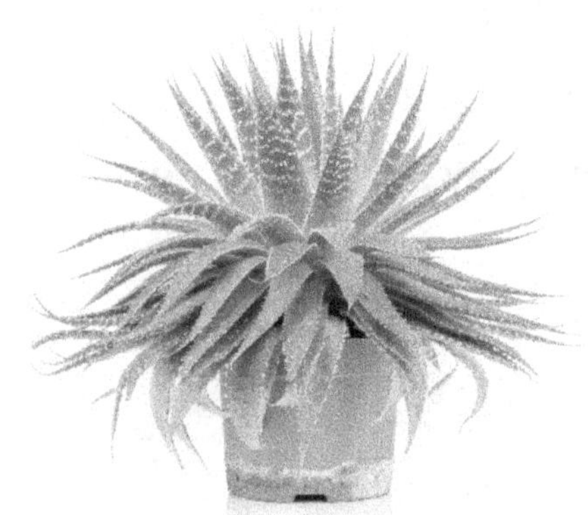

Aloe Vera is a sun-loving succulent that is very easy to care for. It purifies the air of formaldehyde and benzene. It is easy to care for as long as it is getting enough sunlight. It can survive not being watered regularly. Aloe vera is active at night so keep it in a bedroom so that it will be delivering you oxygen while you sleep.

Bamboo Palm

The Bamboo Palm is reported to be the best at filtering toluene, formaldehyde, benzene, trichloroethylene and xylene. In a room with bright light it can grow from 4 to 12 feet tall and 3 to 5 feet wide so make sure you have space for it before you buy it. It likes bright light but is very rugged and can handle low-light conditions as well. Bamboo Palm is really a plant to get excited about if you are improving the indoor air quality of your home or workplace.

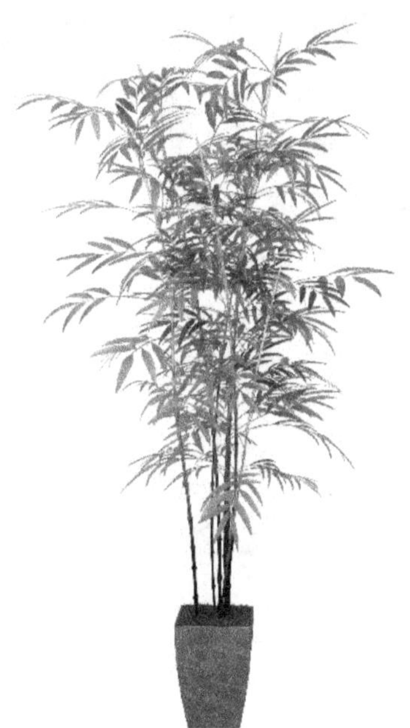

Banana Plant

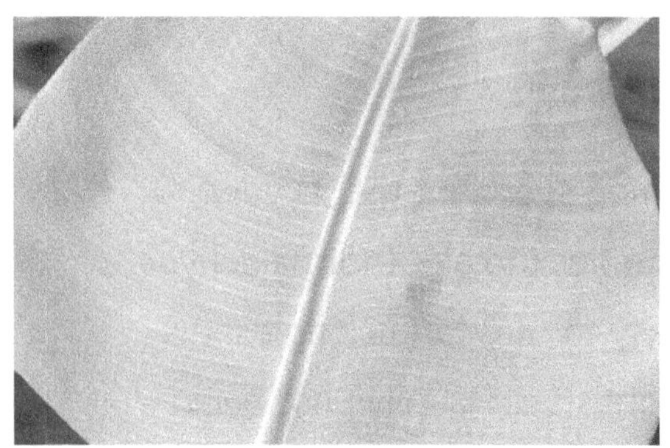

The Banana Plants filter out formaldehyde. And growing a dwarf variety indoors makes for a great conversation piece, as it is rather rare. It has specific needs such as; a large container, a soil pH of 5.5 to 7.0, and 12 hours of bright sunlight a day.

Barberton Daisy

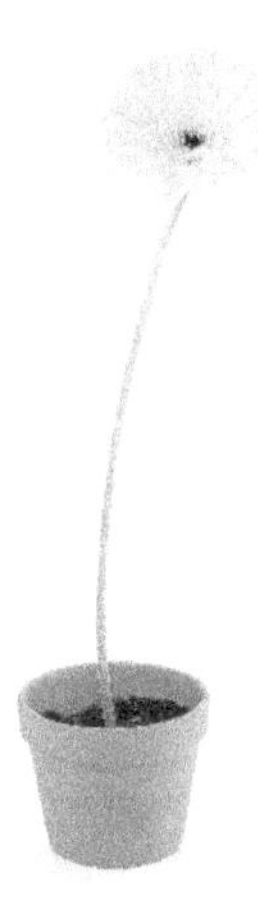

The Barberton Daisy filters out benzene, formaldehyde and trichloroethylene. It is a bit tricky to grow indoors for long periods of time, it is usually purchased and kept for one blooming season and then discarded. To keep one indoors for a long period of time, give it bright light and cool temperatures, below 70F.

Boston Fern

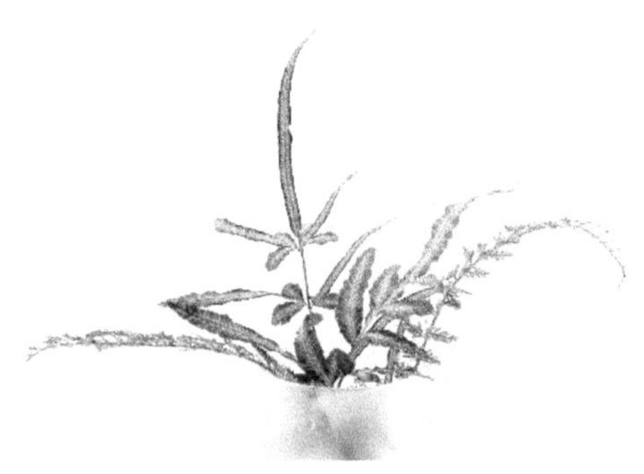

The Boston Fern removes formaldehyde and xylene from the air. It is one of the smaller plants on NASA's list, growing 1 to 3 feet tall and 1 to 4 feet wide. Boston Ferns need bright, indirect light so it should not be put on a windowsill. Keep its soil moist and fertilize once a month.

Chinese Evergreen

The Chinese Evergreen filters out benzene and formaldehyde. For a tropical plant it requires very little maintenance. If you get the soil conditions right, it can handle low light, drought and dry air. Wipe the dust off the leaves occasionally.

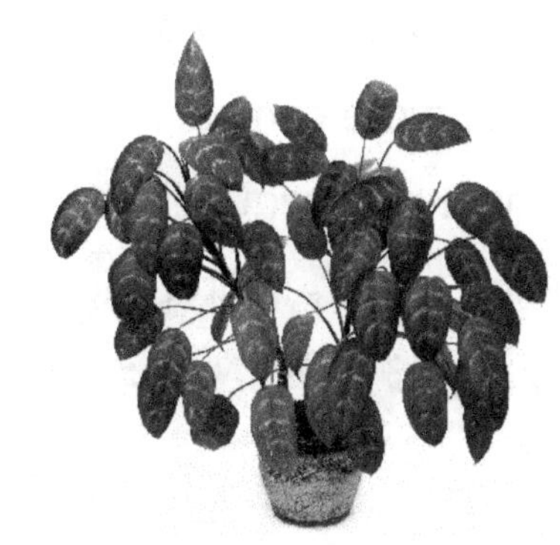

Red-edged Dracaena

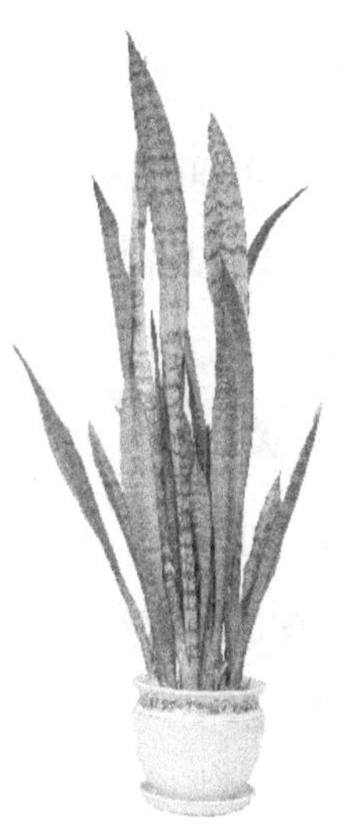

The Red-edged Dracaena is a purifying powerhouse, filtering out formaldehyde, xylene, benzene, and toluene. It is an exciting choice of plant for your home or office. If you are looking for a bold statement for your living room, this shrub can reach 15 feet tall and can tolerate just moderate amounts of light. It can handle many different types of soil, only needs to be watered twice a week and requires little fertilizer.

Variegated Snake Plant

The Snake Plant, also called Mother-in-Laws Tongue, purifies the air of toluene, formaldehyde, trichloroethylene, benzene, xylene. It is a striking plant with multiple, straight leaves that reach upwards so it is great for narrow spaces. It is fantastic for absentee owners, maintaining its good looks through weeks of inattention. They are great for low light, require little fertilizer, have no humidity needs and are fine with normal household temperatures.

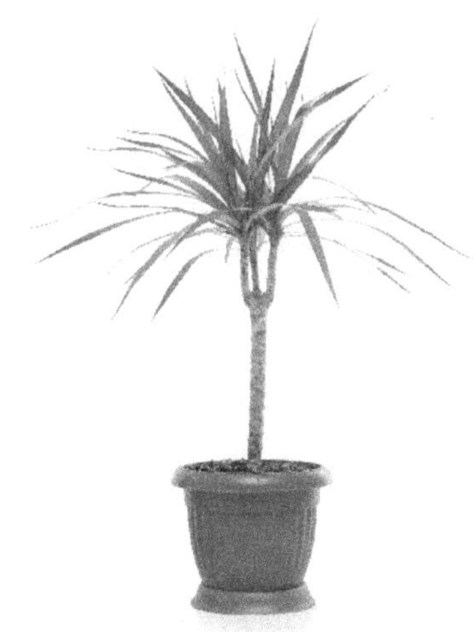

Kimberly Queen Fern

The Kimberly Queen Fern filters formaldehyde, xylene and toluene. It is more compact and tidier than other ferns but has high care requirements. It has needs such as high humidity, bright, indirect light and needs to be watered every 2 to 3 days. Never let the soil dry out completely.

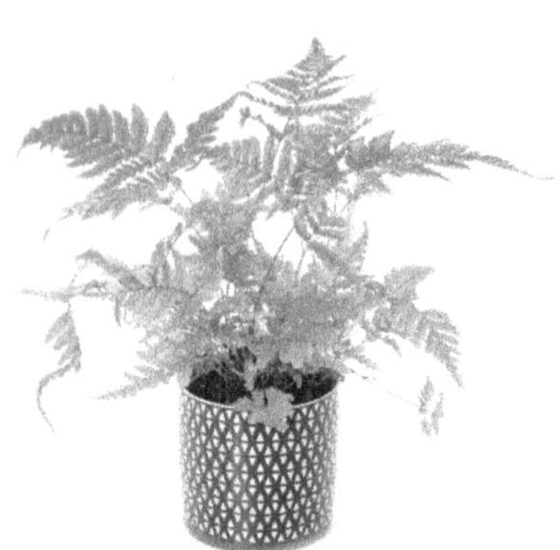

English Ivy

The English Ivy filters out toluene, formaldehyde, xylene, trichloroethylene, benzene, and formaldehyde. It also filters out airborne fecal matter. It is hard to resist having

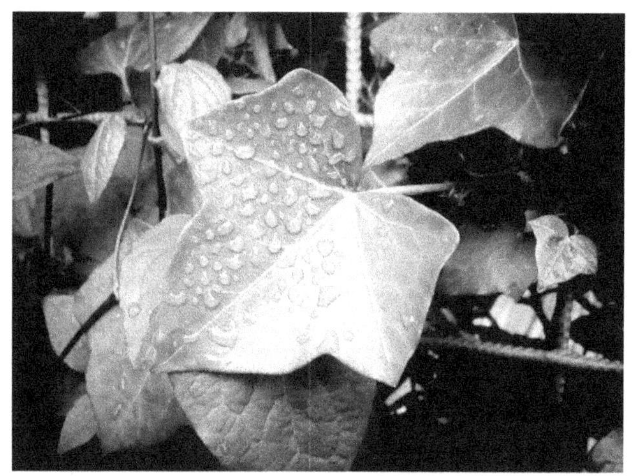

cleaning power like that in your home. It spreads easily and is very low-maintenance and is the most common type of ivy grown indoors. English Ivy needs bright light and should be fertilized once a month.

Florists Chrysanthemum

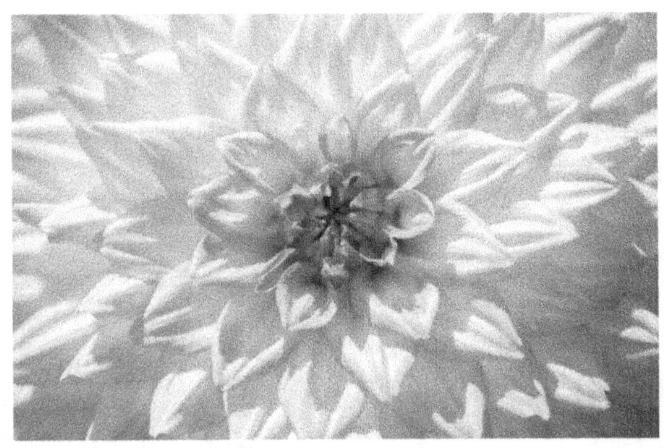

This plant filters out an impressive number of Volatile Organic Compounds, trichloroethylene, benzene, formaldehyde, toluene, xylene and ammonia.

Chrysanthemums are often given as a gift because of their beautiful blooms and low maintenance requirements. They come ready in the right sized pot with the appropriate soil and only need to be watered when the soil feels dry to the touch. They bloom for several weeks and they can be kept after the blooms are spent because of their vibrant foliage.

When choosing to give a Chrysanthemum as a present, you can be sure you have made the right choice as you are providing a loved one with something priceless – clean air.

Janet Craig

Janet Craig is an immensely popular plant in homes and offices, and for good reason. It filters out 3 of the VOCs in the NASA clean air study, formaldehyde, benzene and trichloroethylene.

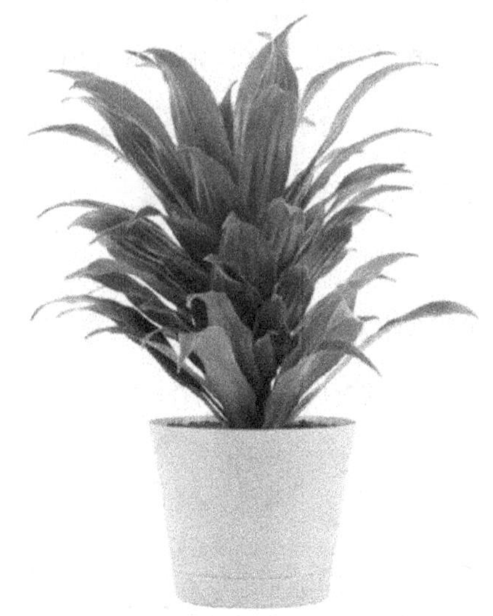

Beyond that impressive claim, Janet Craig is one of the hardiest plants around, tolerating low light and neglect. The plant has no need for humidity and only needs to be fertilized twice a year. When purchasing, be sure that there are between 3 to 5 stalks in one pot, giving the plant a fuller look.

Your Skin Will Give Back to You What You Put In

Our skin is a very vital and complex organ; a strong envelope to keep us intact and everything else out. It is an organ of sensation and touch, closely connected to the great nerve center of our bodies.

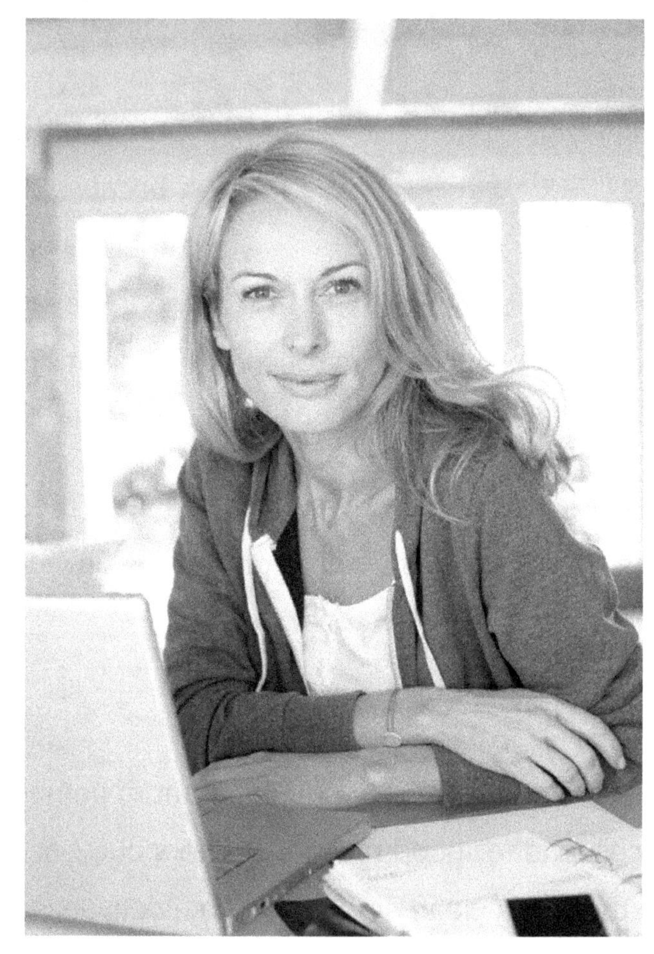

It has many life-preserving functions. It is a temperature regulator because it helps prevent the loss of heat when we are exposed to the cold. In over-heated conditions, the skin relies on tissues helping the heat to escape through profuse sweating. Sweating is also a response to sudden fear or emotional stress.

Our skin maintains its health by excreting sebum, a fatty substance which comes to the surface where it mixes with sweat. This helps keep our skin pliable and moist.

Over-production or underproduction of sebum can cause excessively dry or oily skin. At puberty, the sex hormones affect the skin through the bloodstream and stimulate the sebaceous glands.

The sudden increase of sebum activity may clog the pores and cause blackheads, pimples, or other skin problems. In premature aging, the sebum production slacks off considerably, causing the skin fibers to lose a lot of their elasticity and tone, resulting in dry, leathery looking skin that is wrinkled.

The surface of our skin is also normally acid, and this protective covering is called the acid mantle. It acts as a barrier against any bacterial invasions. If you wash with harsh alkaline type soaps, you will wash off the entire protective acid mantle and it takes quite a lot of hours before the body is able to restore it.

The skin breathes, drawing in oxygen and exhaling impurities, continuing steadily through the day and night.

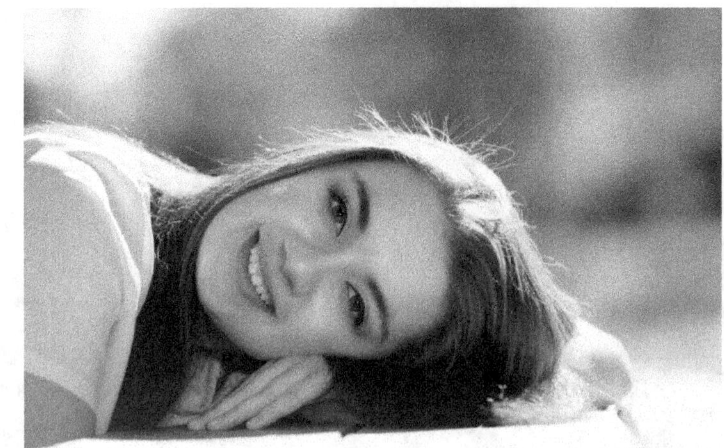

Other toxins are excreted in the form of perspiration which generally collects like tiny beads of droplets on the surface of our skin. Often the skin will take on increased elimination in order to relieve the workload of some distressed organ, like weak kidneys or liver, and even when the lungs are not working adequately.

Toxins from the bowels are sometimes eliminated through the skin too. Were it not for these fantastic arrangements for removing the poisons from the body, the blood would become so polluted it would not even be able to support our life.

Another function nature has given to the skin is the ability to absorb certain external substances such as ointments or lotions that are applied to it. This absorption also means that unless the skin is properly bathed and cared for, the impurities deposited on the surface through perspiration accumulate and the waste may be absorbed in the body, causing the skin to become toxic.

Our skin consists of four layers which are constantly being renewed. The surface layer which is the epidermis flakes off and depends upon the layers underneath for constant renewal. That is why it is so important to use a little friction when bathing so that the dead flaking cells can be thoroughly removed. We also need to use cosmetics sparingly, taking care never to apply fresh makeup over the stale makeup.

Dry Brushing

Dry brushing has many benefits. When you do dry brushing, you brush towards the heart, starting with your feet and hands. It is an excellent anti-aging skin care method that supports lymphatic drainage, it exfoliates your skin, keeping it soft, and it cleans the pores of your skin, and reduces cellulite, giving you a natural energy boost. Dermatologists agree that gently brushing the skin rates similarly to massage, which has well-documented benefits.

Even though we might look after our skin, there are problems that we can experience such as brown spots, acne, eczema and other skin disorders.

Brown spots

The appearance of brown spots on the hands and face is a cosmetic problem that affects many older men and women. Different methods of removing these tell-tale aging signs have been used by many people. An old-time favorite remedy is castor oil which is rubbed onto the brown spots every night until they disappear. Some sources recommend external applications of fresh juice from some ground up parsley.

Acne

Perhaps no skin diseases cause people so much distress as acne. Cleanliness and nutrition are extremely important in preventing this unpleasant skin disorder. Diets which are high in fat content stimulate the sebaceous glands. The increased activity forces oil to the surface where they often get clogged which results in pimples and acne. Doctors will often recommend retinol products for treating acne, but in discovering that, they also discovered how effective it has proved against wrinkles.

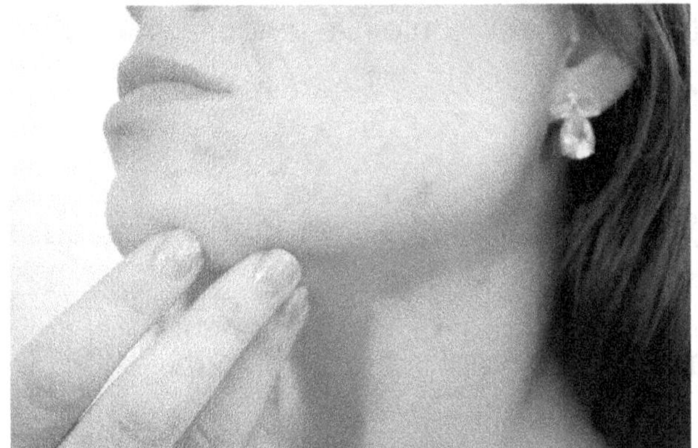

Eczema and psoriasis

If you add fatty acids to your diet, you can greatly improve the conditions of eczema. Unsaturated fatty acids have also been found to have huge beneficial effects on the skin disorder, psoriasis. What are the ideal fatty acids to add to your diet? Omega 3 is the one.

Even though aging is a natural process of growing older there are still many factors that play a role in whether we will age faster than our biological age, or whether we will grow old gracefully. A lot of people do look older than they really are because they do things that advance the aging process. Look at these factors that can cause you to age prematurely:

Attitude

The mind sure does play a role in whether we will age slower or faster. Happier people look younger, always. When you hope, have optimism, joy, and contentment in your life, youthful vigor exudes from the face and body. Studies prove that happier people live longer with fewer health problems.

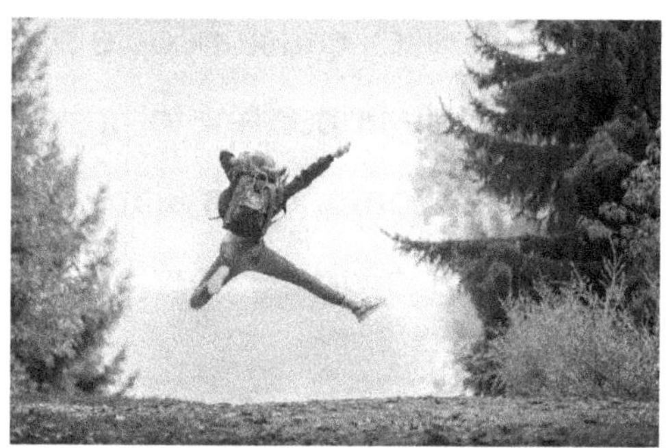

Continual anger and stress etches itself in the skin causing deep lines and wrinkles. How your body and face reveal your emotions and expressions can determine how prematurely you develop wrinkles on your skin.

Smoking and drinking

When you smoke and drink in excess, you are not doing your skin any good, because these two habits deplete your body of necessary nutrients. The skin requires much collagen, elastin, and hydration to look youthful and healthy. If you smoke, you deprive your entire body of oxygen.

Drinking, too, can leave permanent marks on your body. Not only are you damaging your kidney and liver, but facial skin can become discolored over time. There are 4 aging things that smoking, and drinking bring to your skin: Dehydration, swelling, collagen depletion, and inflammation.

Cold, Sun, and Moisture

It is so easy to accelerate the aging process just simply by basking in the sun's rays.

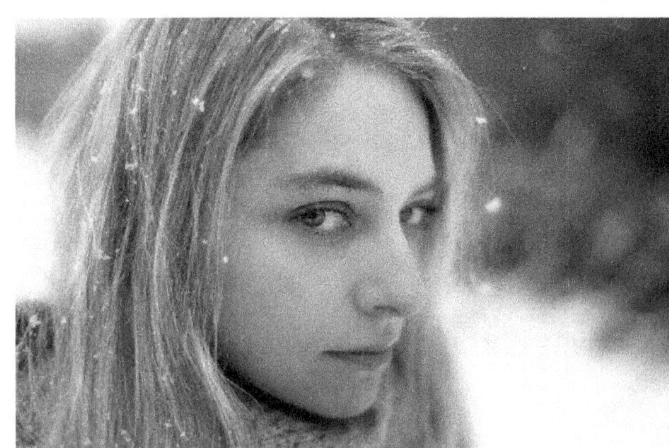

Damage caused by the sun is the top cause of wrinkles.

Age spots, too, and other discoloration forms worsen under the harmful UV rays of the sun. Someone who has spent years working on their tan will ultimately end up with leathery and wrinkled skin.

Once you extend your time in the sun over 20 minutes, the benefits that you would receive from taking in some essential vitamin D are all counteracted by the UV rays damage to your skin. Cold weather too, is just as dangerous, causing thin, wrinkled skin. If you have acne and you use harsh treatments that deplete your skin of natural oils, you damage its natural elasticity.

Diet

Food has a huge impact on the skin. When you choose foods high in sugar and fat, i.e. processed foods, with few vegetables and fruit, you create something inside your body that goes completely against anti-aging methods. When you replace all that 'bad food' with foods that are healthy and organic, you avoid creating inflammation from building up in your body which is one big aging factor.

Weight

If you are not at a normal weight, you probably are too heavy or too thin. Being too overweight or too underweight adds years on to the aging process. Being underweight, you will lose the natural fats in your face, resulting in sagging skin; jowls and wrinkles.

Not even a facelift or Botox treatments can help a thin and underweight face to replace the natural youthful fattiness that used to fill out your face in earlier days. When you add on a couple of extra pounds to a very underweight body, you can make yourself look softer and more wrinkle-free.

Too much weight creates the appearance of being older than you are because you have poor muscle tone. People who are overweight become less active as they age. Because of all that inactivity, they create for themselves chronic health problems like diabetes and heart disease.

Malnourishing your body can add on anything from 10 to 20 years to your appearance and health. It is never too late to fix things. A rich diet that is full of antioxidants, fresh and natural foods and plenty of muscle building exercises can kick-start your metabolism again.

If you are serious about your weight and trying to reverse some aging habits, it might be a good start to see a nutritionist periodically so they work out a high energy, age-fight low fat program for you to adhere to.

Choices

Every day we make choices that will hinder or delay or help the process of aging. You should involve yourself in regular workouts to keep your body looking toned, healthy, and full of energy. It's your choice to opt for the television set with your

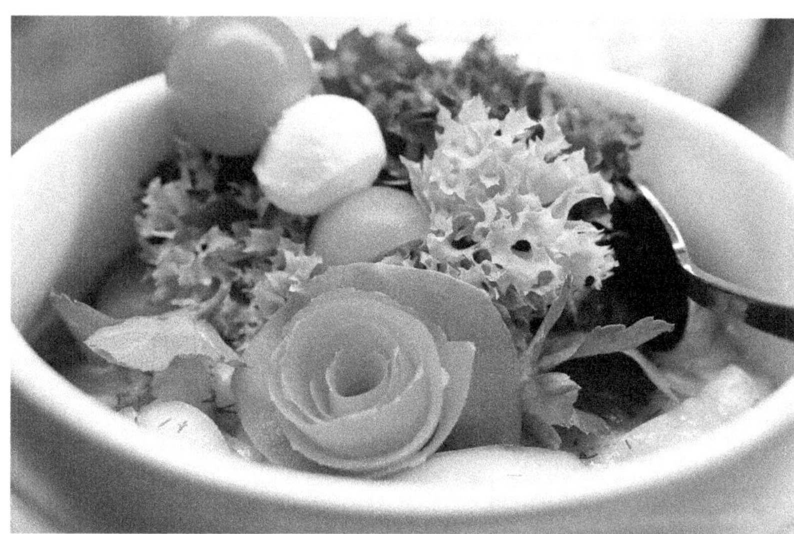

bowl of chips or it's your choice to get 'out there', exercising and building your body for a youthful and more disease-free body.

When you make the right choice to work for your body and not against it, you help the anti-aging process big time. That means listening to your body and what it is telling you. Don't just carry on eating when you are full. Rest when you are tired. Focus on your body's needs, turning towards natural inventions and natural interventions rather than the chemical solutions, if you want to turn back the hands of time. Because these choices to work with your body and its natural rhythms will pay you back in dividends that you would never have dreamed of.

Stress

Stress, unfortunately, is a very good recipe for aging. And we all suffer from time to

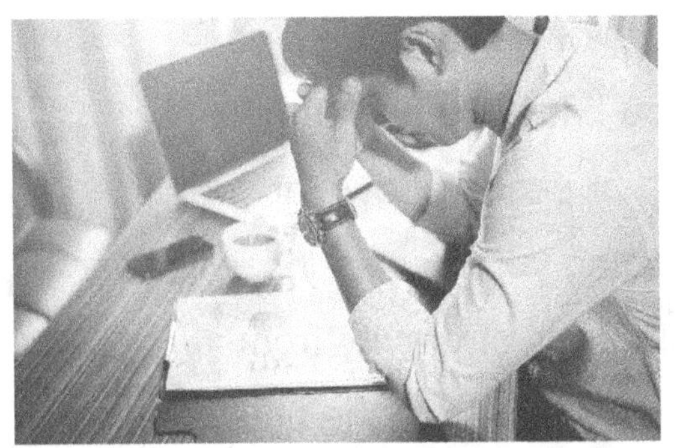

time. Chronic stress can ruin your health and your mental state too, which is a top aging factor.

All those worries, frowns, and negative feelings encourage the aging process. It's not that easy just to say, get rid of stress, but it is necessary to find ways to de-stress like a wonderful massage, calming and natural herbs, foods that de-stress and certainly exercise.

We all know that those late nights, the early starts, the work stress, drinking the night before, lots of sugar – all this FOMO takes a major toll on your skin. When you can't bear to miss a party, to watch every hot Netflix movie, or try every new cocktail bar, busily spending hours on social media to keep your friends updated, it all takes its toll.

In your 20s, you are probably too busy to see the warning signs coming. But they are all adding up to premature aging of your body, your health, and your skin. By the time you hit your 30s, you can expect to be starting to see the results, dry eyes, sagging skin, puffy and red face, wrinkles, dry hair …. The list will get longer over time. Nobody said there's anything wrong with aging, its life's natural process but if you don't look after your body and skin, you might just be 'old' 20 years ahead of your time.

Spend too Much Time on Social Media

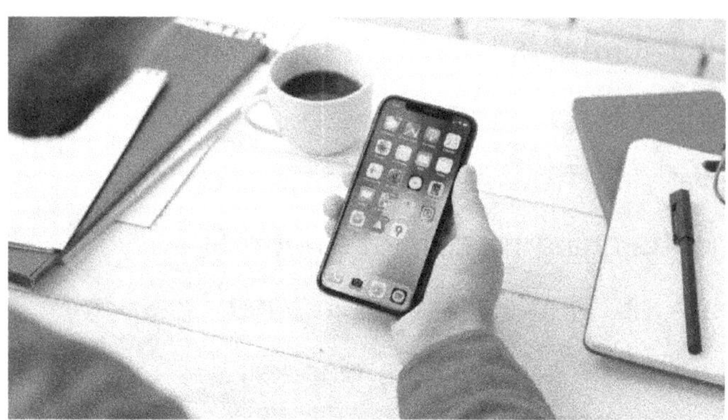

Ever heard of 'tech-neck'? It can cause you back and neck problems with all that peering down at your phone, aging your neck and jawline faster. The pull of gravity from looking downwards all the time means sagging in the lower face starting earlier than it should.

Lying in Bed Using your Phone

All that bright light from your phone screen or laptop can certainly hamper your sleep – let alone the damage you do to your eyes when you stare at that bright light in a dark room as well. It can definitely cause dry eyes and eye infections because your blinking mechanism is all suppressed.

Computer Lighting

When you spend too long staring at your computer or television, it's a no-no when it comes to trying to keep a youthful skin. The light, known as high energy visible light can break down elastin and skin collagen structures that are responsible for keeping your skin youthful and firm.

Drinking too Much

A big negative side-effect of drinking too much alcohol is it dries out the skin. It acts as a diuretic too, causing your skin to become dehydrated and flaky.

Not Sleeping Enough

When you don't get enough sleep, or you don't drink enough water, you can wake up with puffy skin and even extra makeup will not take that away. When you don't get your 40 winks every day, your face can start looking pale and lifeless.

Turning the Heat Up

When you are cold you want to be warm, but over-hot temperatures can dry out the skin caused by central heating. Combinations of hot and cold weather are harsh on the skin leading to dry, sallow and dull complexions caused by dehydration. People need 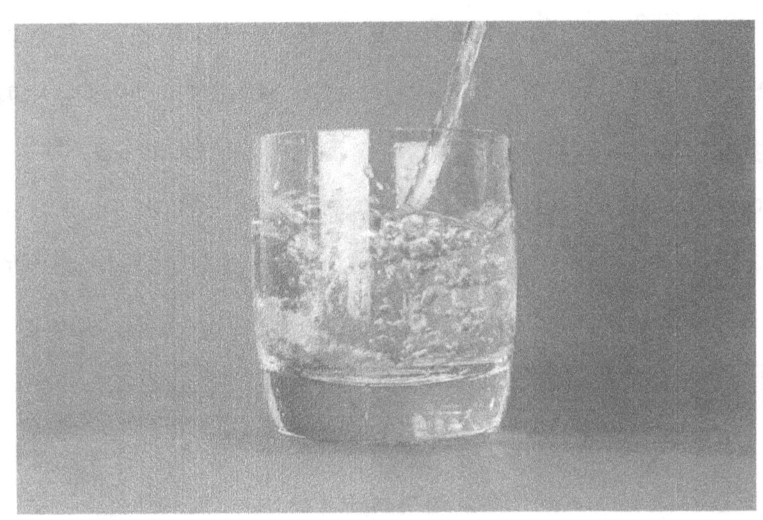 to realize that drinking water in winter is just as important as in the summer.

Sleeping on the Wrong Bed Linens

Did you know that the wrong kind of bed linen can add lines to your face? Ideally, what you are looking for are soft, pillowcases made from silk, so much gentler on the skin, and particularly if you are someone who likes to sleep on your side. Pillowcases that are made from synthetic materials can result in small folds and creases on your face and body which, over time, develop into premature wrinkling, say the skin experts.

Eating Unhealthily - or Not Eating Enough

It should not be a surprise to anyone that sugary, oily foods aren't going to do your skin any good. When you are too busy in your life to maintain a healthy lifestyle and eat nutritional foods, you accelerate the volume loss from your face.

Detox Your Body for Healthy Skin

A detox is an excellent idea to benefit your skin. You feel wonderful and you look younger. There are certain superfoods that are packed with nutrients to get your skin in reverse again. When you detox, you are not starving yourself, it really means cleansing your body from all the toxins that have built up from the consumption of too many processed foods. The body naturally detoxes all the time but when you incorporate a detox regime into your life you put that natural process to its maximum benefits. Including these foods into your diet, you are going to notice stuff happening, very good stuff, inside and out:

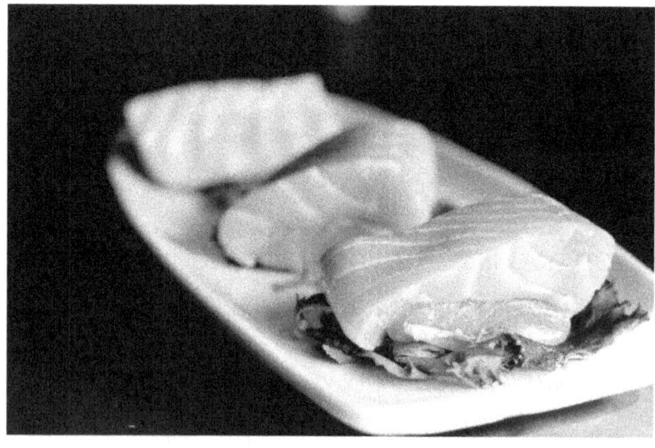

Fresh Fish (e.g., sardines, salmon, tilapia)

Fish truly has health benefits, which is why fish forms a big part in most anti-aging diets. Reason being, they have such high levels of omega-3 fatty acids in them and plenty of essential vitamins that are proven to make people healthier and younger looking.

Herbal Tea (e.g., green tea, black tea, peppermint tea)

Herbal teas detoxify the body which is ideal for an anti-aging diet. They are safe and easy to use, to help you look younger from the inside out. They act as purifiers, helping to fight bacteria, cleanse impurities from your body and heal broken skin or wounds.

Tart Cherry Juice

Drinking **Traverse Bay Farms tart cherry juice** daily is a great way to keep you skin healthy. The reason is tart cherries are packed full of power anthocyanins. This is a natural anti-inflammatory to help keep inflammation in check. Also, tart cherries are nature's leading source of naturally occurring melatonin for healthy sleep.

Greens (e.g., spinach, broccoli, Swiss chard, basil, etc.)

No anti-aging diet would work without leafy greens, because they are so detoxifying. They supply all the necessary vitamins and minerals to look younger. When you are short of iron you become tired, particularly for the older woman, and which can be so easily remedied by taking more vegetables. Look younger because your blood is clean and healthy.

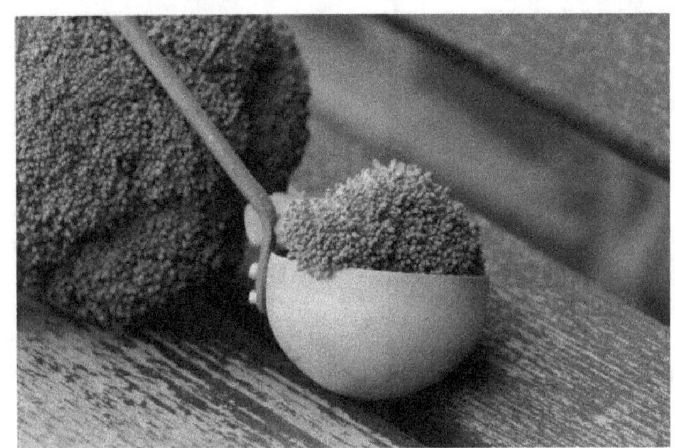

Citrus (e.g., limes, lemons, oranges, grapefruit)

These fruits make you look younger because they supply abundant antioxidants, to fight off free radicals that accelerate getting old. Citrus fruits flush out the intestines, clearing your body of bacteria and toxins and keeping your body hydrated.

Pineapples

Pineapples contain bromelain, enzymes for digestive health because they clean out your colon. Pineapples have been used for hundreds of years for digestion problems.

Conclusion

By adding the above, you also need to take away. That means taking away refined sugars, processed foods, alcohol, excessive eggs, and dairy and meat. You need to be consistent in the process of natural anti-aging skin care because then only will it be a beautiful canvas that tells your story of love and care.

Resources:

YumsUp.com

- Step-by-step recipes videos to make great tasting recipes for every meal of the day.

- **Website:** YumsUp.com

Traverse Bay Farms

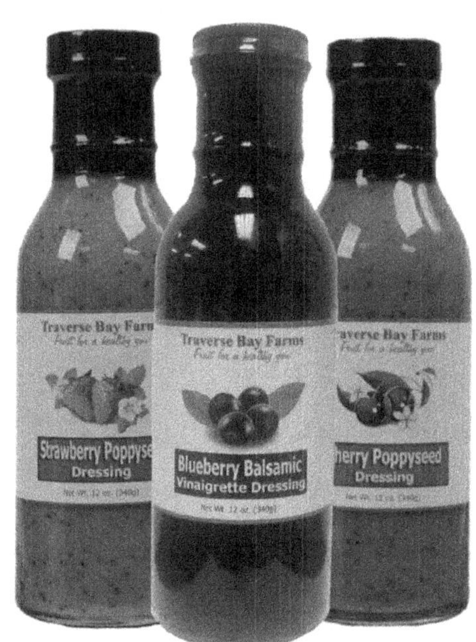

- Winner of 30+ national food awards at America's largest and most competitive food competitions. #1 nationally award-winning superfood company in America.

  Complete selection of all national salsa, fruit-based barbecue sauces, jams, jellies and more.

  No-added sugar dried cherries, chocolate-covered dried cherries, strawberries, blueberries and more.

  Cherry juice concentrate to healthy joints and more. If you're looking for all-natural products, check out Traverse Bay Farms.

- **Website:** TraverseBayFarms.com

Health Smart Recipes

- How-to Recipes and Information.

- **Website:** HealthSmartRecipes.com